For more copies of *Stroke*, **write to:**

PRITCHETT & HULL ASSOCIATES, INC.
3440 OAKCLIFF RD NE STE 110
ATLANTA GA 30340-3006

or call toll free: 800-241-4925

Stroke

Early Stages of Recovery

This book is written to help you understand stroke. It should not be used to replace any of your health team's advice or treatment.

Table of Contents

Introduction

Strokes often happen without warning, suddenly changing your world. If you or someone close to you has had a stroke, you may feel afraid and confused. You may wonder:

- ► What are the chances for survival after stroke?
- ► How big is this stroke?
- ► How will the stroke change me, or our loved ones?
- ► How long will it take to get better?

It is hard to answer these questions because each person is different. A stroke can range from mild to severe. How much or how soon a person recovers depends on many things. For a while, you may not know how fast or how much recovery will happen.

This book describes how strokes occur and the early stages of recovery. You will find out why someone with a stroke acts the way he does and what may happen as he gets better.

If you had a stroke, you may not read this book until after you are well on your way to recovery. It will help you understand what has happened and how loved ones can support each other. You will also learn ways you might help yourself along this journey. Remember, the family takes this journey together, even if only one of you had the stroke.

Much comfort can be found in knowing what is going on. If you have questions, ask them. Understanding stroke and having a positive outlook will help you through this time.

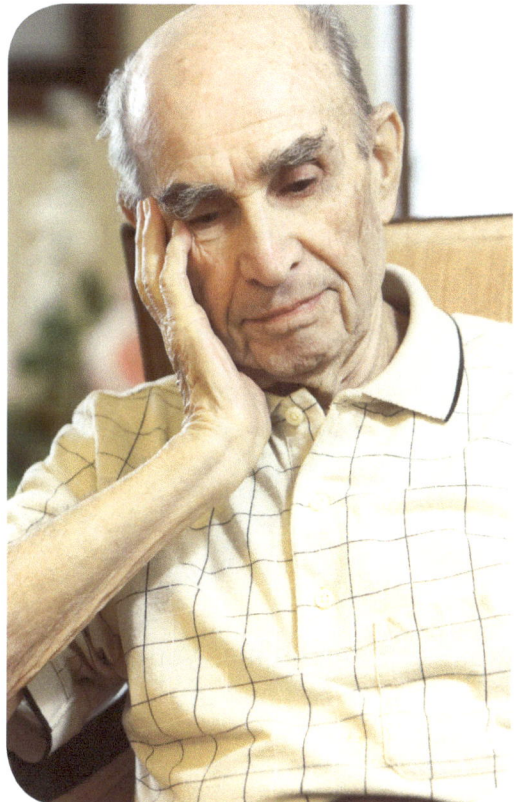

What is a stroke?

Your brain is the control center for your whole body. It lets you see, hear, taste, smell, feel, think and move around. Each area has special tasks to do, and some areas work together to get their jobs done.

When your heart beats, it sends blood through arteries and veins to every part of your body. Blood carries oxygen to brain cells through arteries in and around the brain. Oxygen keeps the brain cells alive and working well.

When the brain's blood flow stops or leaks into the wrong place, brain cells in that area die. This is called a **stroke** or **cerebral vascular accident** (CVA). Brain cells which die will not recover (permanent brain damage). Other brain cells are in shock and will start working again after a while. No one can tell just how long it will take for these cells to begin working again. Most healing happens in the first year, but people may improve their skills for much longer. Also, people may learn new skills to replace the ones they've lost.

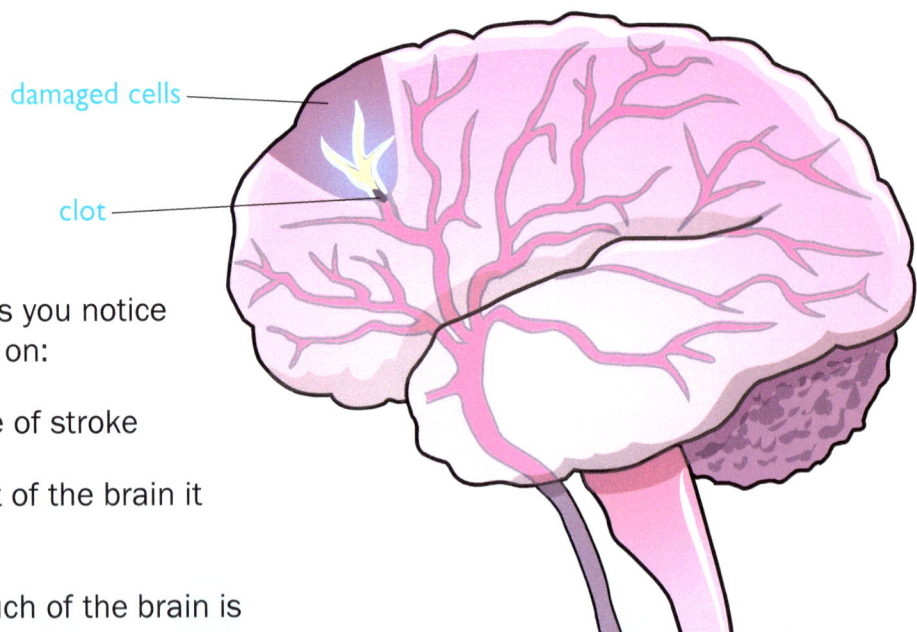

damaged cells

clot

The changes you notice will depend on:

▶ the type of stroke

▶ the part of the brain it harms

▶ how much of the brain is harmed

Warning signs of a stroke:

- ► sudden numbness or weakness on one side of your body

- ► sudden changes in vision, especially in one eye

- ► trouble speaking or understanding what you hear

- ► sudden severe headache of unknown cause

- ► trouble walking or staying balanced

These signs can last from ten minutes to hours. **If you have any of these, call 911 at once*. Early care can prevent permanent damage.**

If any of these signs happen and then go away, it may be a **transient ischemic attack** or **TIA.**

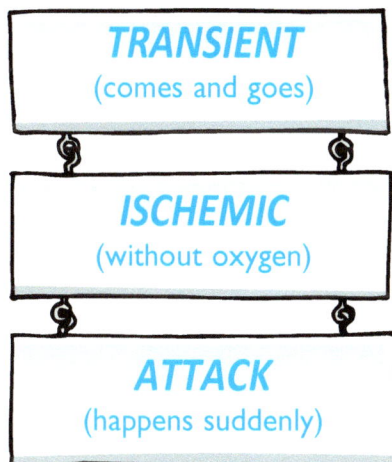

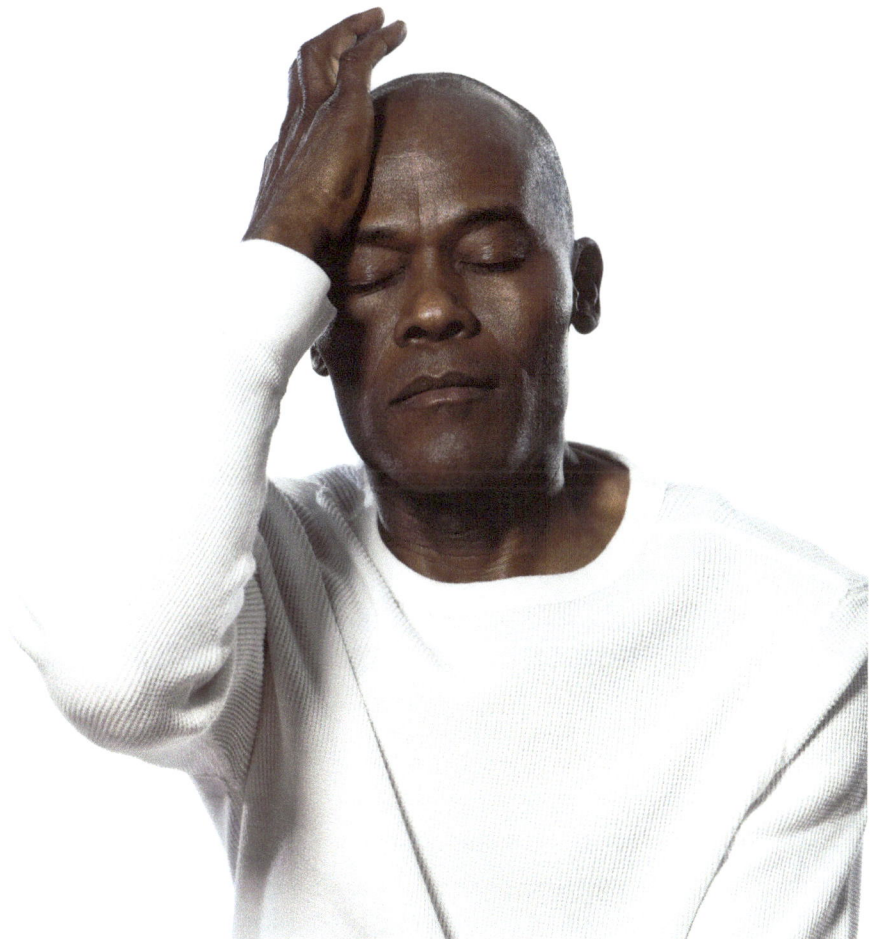

TRANSIENT
(comes and goes)

ISCHEMIC
(without oxygen)

ATTACK
(happens suddenly)

* If 911 is not available in your area, go to the nearest hospital.

Types of stroke:

Not all strokes are alike. The type of stroke depends on how it happens:

Ischemic (too little blood flow):

embolism
Sometimes the heart or blood vessels in the neck release a blood clot that travels through arteries. Clots can float through big arteries with no problem. If a clot tries to pass through small arteries in the brain, it gets stuck and blocks the flow of blood. This type of stroke is called a cerebral embolism.

thrombosis
Another type of stroke happens when a brain artery clogs up. Fatty buildup (plaque) collects inside an artery wall. As blood flows through the artery, it sticks to the plaque's rough edges and builds up a clot. Over time, this can build a dam in the artery that stops blood flow. Brain cells on the other side can't get oxygen and die.

Hemorrhagic (too much blood flow):

hemorrhage
A hemorrhage happens when a blood vessel in the brain breaks open. Blood spills out and damages the brain cells near the injured blood vessel. The broken vessel no longer carries blood, and further brain damage results. Sometimes this is caused by a "bubble" that bursts in a blood vessel, called an aneurysm.

Embolism

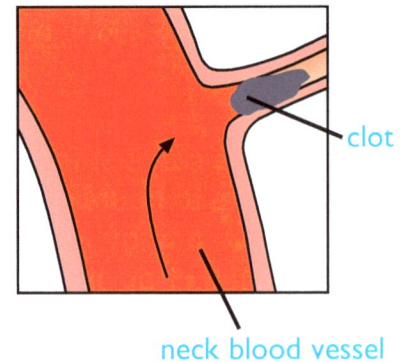

clot

neck blood vessel

Thrombosis

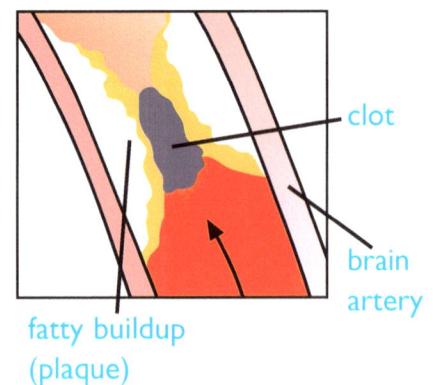

clot

brain artery

fatty buildup (plaque)

Hemorrhage

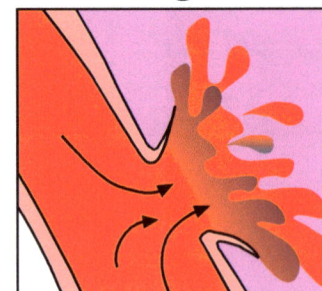

Parts of the brain

A stroke can damage the brain on either the right or left side. Sometimes a stroke happens deep inside the brain near the center. It may help to know a little about what these parts of the brain do. Then you will understand some of the changes that you may experience.

Right Brain

- feels and moves left side of body
- controls emotions
- organizes
- keeps track of time
- pays attention to the left side of space

Left Brain

- feels and moves right side of body
- controls speech
- understands language
- reads, writes, does math
- remembers words

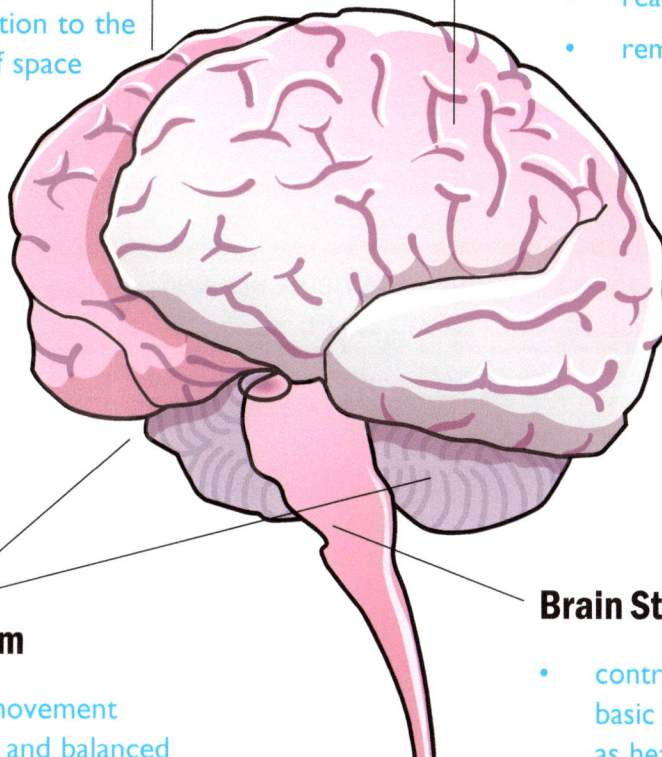

Cerebellum

- keeps movement smooth and balanced

Brain Stem

- controls and regulates basic body functions such as heartbeat, breathing, swallowing and blinking
- controls alertness
- focuses attention

Hospital arrival

As soon as you get to the hospital, doctors will run tests to discover the cause of the stroke. They will learn where and how much damage has happened from the stroke. The tests may include:

► **MRI Scan** *(Magnetic Resonance Imaging)*
a special Xray which gives pictures of the brain so that areas with damage can be seen.

CT Scan

► **CT Scan** *(Computerized Tomography)*
a scan which also gives pictures of the brain to show any damage. Only certain kinds of strokes are seen on CT scans.

► **Duplex Scan**
a test that uses ultrasound waves to make pictures of the carotid artery (the main artery taking blood to the brain).

► **Echocardiogram** *(echo)*
a test to find out if an opening in the heart allowed a blood clot to pass through to the brain.

► **Angiogram**
dye is placed in blood vessels to look at blood flow to the brain.

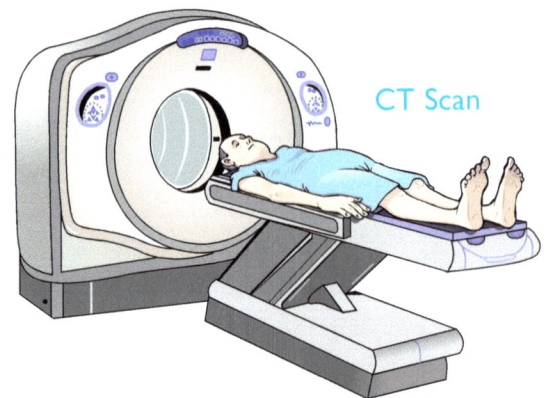

If the stroke is caused by a blood clot, you may receive medicine (antithrombotic) to dissolve the clot. This medicine is given within the first few hours of a stroke. Other kinds of strokes may need surgery to repair blood vessels or remove extra blood or fluid. A "thrombectomy" removes a blood clot from the artery.

Early Care Guide for Families

Your loved one may spend time in the Intensive Care Unit (ICU). While there, he or she is watched for any changes, and treatments are done to help prevent more damage to the brain.

Your loved one may be unconscious and not able to speak or make any willful response. He may hold his arms and legs stiffly in one position or they may seem to be very relaxed and heavy. There may be splints on his arms or legs. If he is moving around a lot in bed, he may be softly tied with cloth restraints. The ties may upset you, but they keep him safe. They can prevent a confused person from pulling out tubes or falling out of bed.

Visitors may be limited during this time. The nurses will tell you when you can visit and how long you can stay. Use the time between visits to prepare yourself and your loved ones for the next few days and weeks.

Family tips:

► It is OK to gently touch and speak to the person. It may seem strange to touch and talk to someone who can't react, but this can comfort him.

► Talk to your loved one in a soothing tone using normal speech. Calmly tell him where he is and what has happened. It may help to remind him of the day and time.

► Give a list of your personal or household needs to a good friend or family member. Ask for help with errands, child care, yard work, meals and household chores.

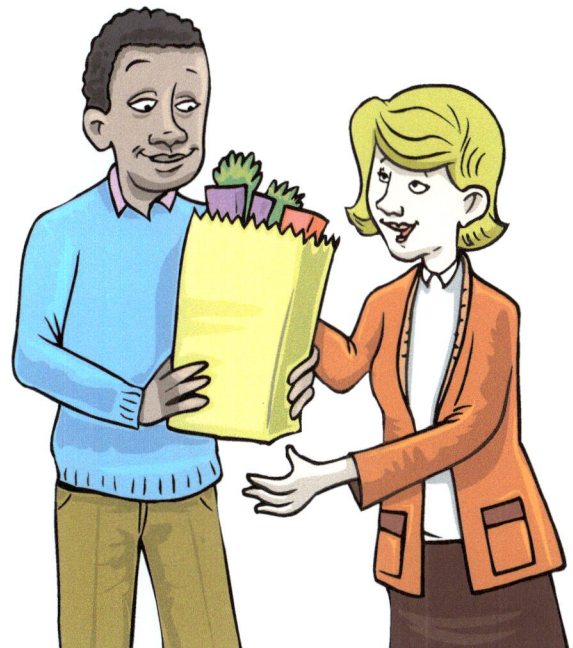

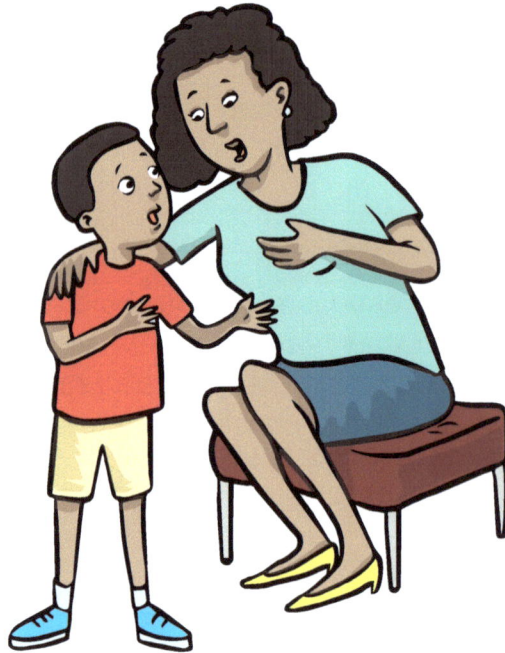

► Young children may be upset by the stroke but not show it until later. Explain what has happened in a way they can understand.

► Find an easy way to let others know of your loved one's progress. Leave a voice message on your phone, or ask a friend to post updates on an internet site for you. Then you won't wear yourself out giving the same information over and over.

► Prepare friends ahead of time for the changes in how the person looks and acts. Some people feel awkward around hospitals but do fine once they know what to expect.

► This early stage after the stroke can be an emotional roller coaster for you. This is normal. While in this stage, let others know how you feel. Think of them as your support system. They may be family members, close friends, your doctor, co-workers, clergy or anyone who can listen to your feelings and offer a helping hand.

► Take care of yourself by resting and not skipping meals.

Hospital Stay

Once the critical stage has passed, you or your loved one may need to stay in the hospital for a while. During this time you will learn more about effects of the stroke. Learn all you can so that everyone will be ready when you leave the hospital.

Family tips:

► Make the hospital room seem more like home. Bring in a few favorite things such as a pillow, blanket, posters and photos of family, friends or pets. Label photos with names and dates.

► Responses may be slow and not consistent. Bring up only one idea at a time. Use short, simple sentences, and give plenty of time to respond.

► Keep a large calendar and clock in view to keep up with the date and time. Mark off each passing day.

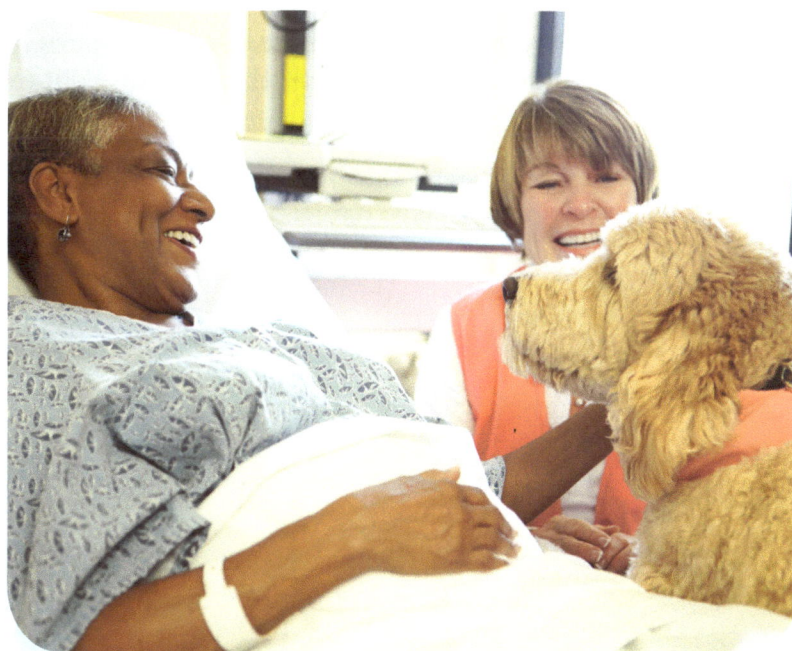

► Give a lot of encouragement and praise.

Getting Organized

It's normal to feel confused and overwhelmed during this time. When a sudden health change happens, there are many decisions to be made. A helper, or "advocate" will be needed during the hospital stay and afterward.

Family tips:

► Now is a good time to talk with your hospital service coordinator about money matters. He or she may ask you for other insurance information.

► Learn about your loved one's insurance. You may find that some needs are not covered. If necessary, get help in calling the insurance company to ask for special consideration.

► If the patient is too young for Social Security benefits, he may qualify for Social Security Disability Income (SSDI). Also, find out if he has a disability or long-term care policy through his workplace. Ask your service coordinator to help you understand these complicated financial matters and fill out needed forms.

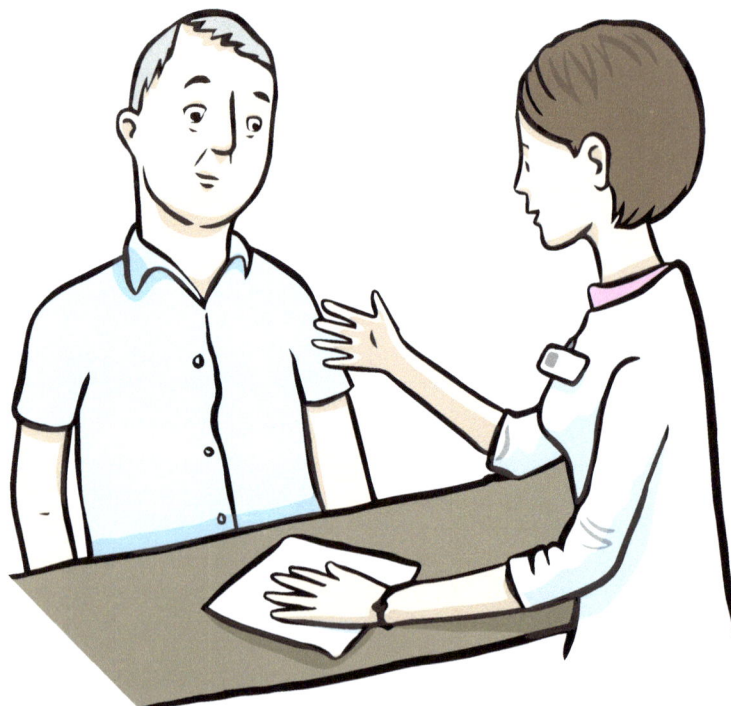

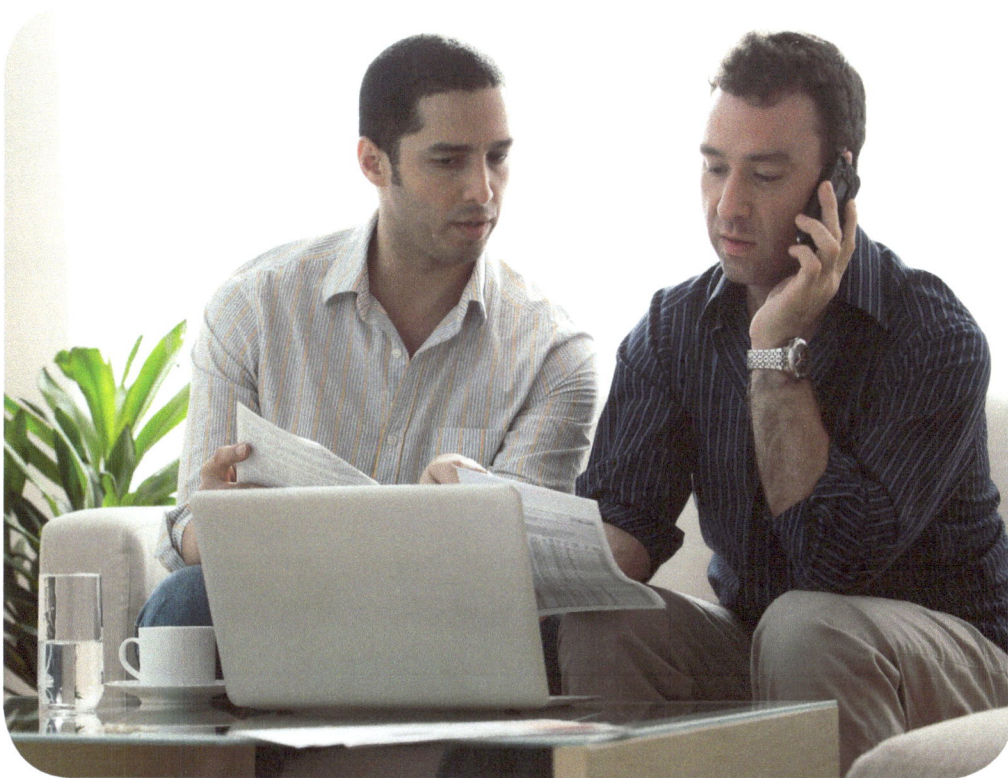

▶ Many friends and family members can help. Each will have a different talent. Some might be helpful with money or insurance issues. Others may be comfortable helping out in the hospital room. Let them help in whatever way is best for them and for you.

▶ Get a file box to save medical and financial papers during this journey. You may need them down the road.

▶ Keep notes of any questions you may have.

Service Coordinator:

Gathers facts about the patient's life and family as well as financial and emotional needs, helps with discharge plans and gives support and guidance. Some hospitals call this person a case manager or social worker.

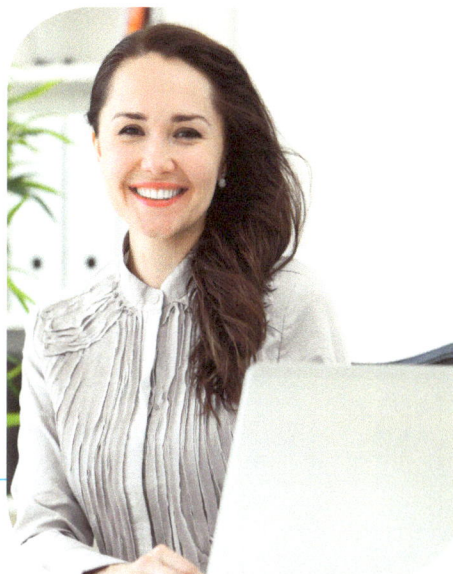

Changes

A stroke can cause changes in how a person:

► moves

► communicates

► eats, drinks and swallows

► controls his bladder and bowels

► senses (sight, touch, position)

► acts

► thinks

Accept the fact that you can't force a person to get well faster by doing (or not doing) certain things. Having caring people around helps a lot, but recovery has its own time frame. **Focus on goals instead of time deadlines.**

Movement

A stroke often changes the way a person moves. Some people have a lot of change while others have very little.

A stroke on one side of the brain can cause **muscle weakness** on the other side of the body. Weakness may be mild (hemi-paresis), or it may keep the person from moving the affected limbs at all (hemiplegia). Joints can then become stiff and tight. If face, mouth, neck and throat muscles are weak, the face may droop. This may cause drooling from one side of the mouth. It may also cause slurred speech (dysarthria) or swallowing problems (dysphagia).

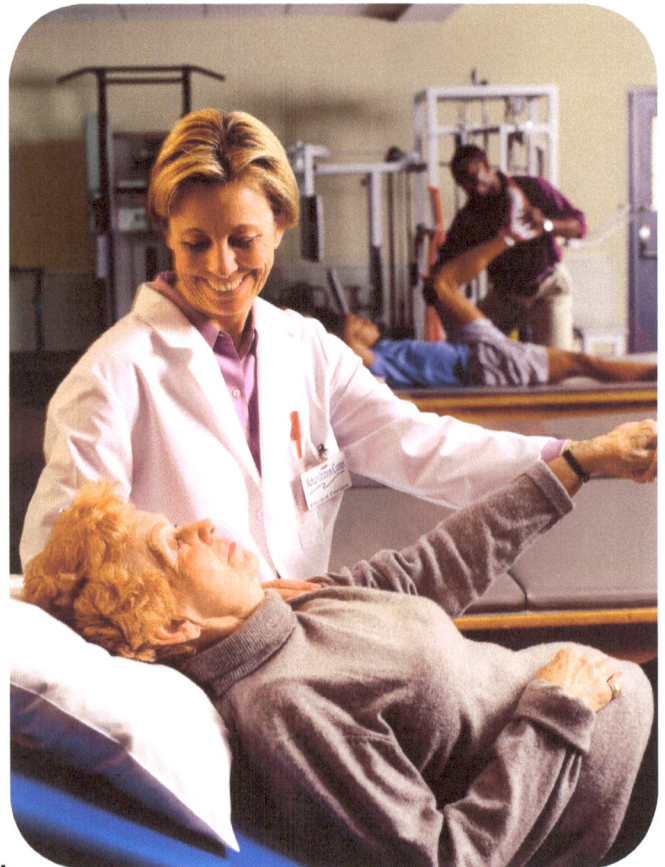

The brain sends signals to muscles to make them tense or relax. After a stroke, the signals can change. Parts of the body may feel limp and heavy or become tight. Changes in **muscle tone** often make it hard to control movement.

Muscles work together to make smooth movements. Some strokes can cause jerky movements (ataxia) or problems with coordination.

Physical and occupational therapists (see page 17) can teach you and your loved one how to improve movement after stroke.

Family tips:

▶ Find out what your loved one can do for himself, and help with only what is needed. He will relearn faster if he tries to do things on his own.

▶ Encourage the person to use his weak arms and legs as much as he can for such things as grooming, dressing and eating. Sometimes the therapist may restrain the strong limbs as a way to increase movement of the weaker ones. This allows the brain to send messages to the weaker side: "you can do it!"

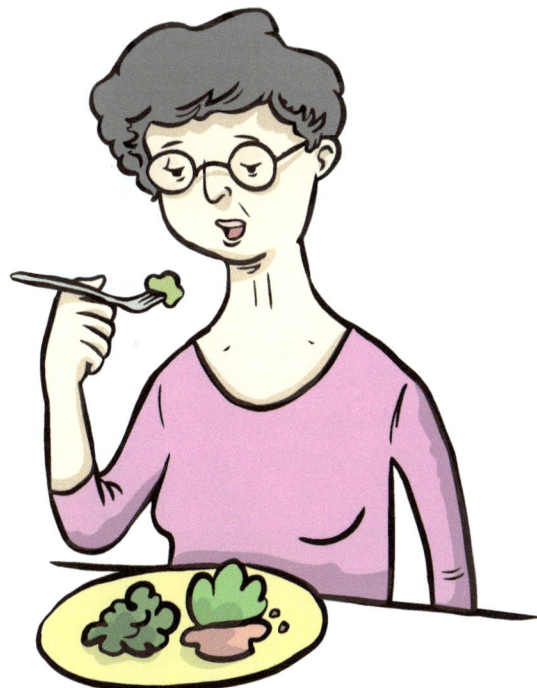

► Learn exercises to stretch out tight joints and improve strength and coordination. Exercising at home will be important.

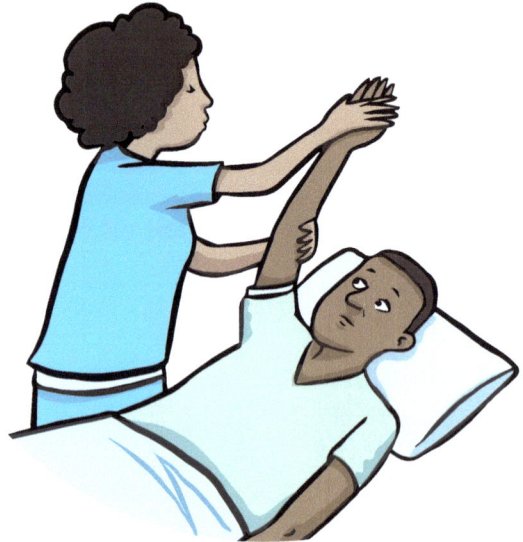

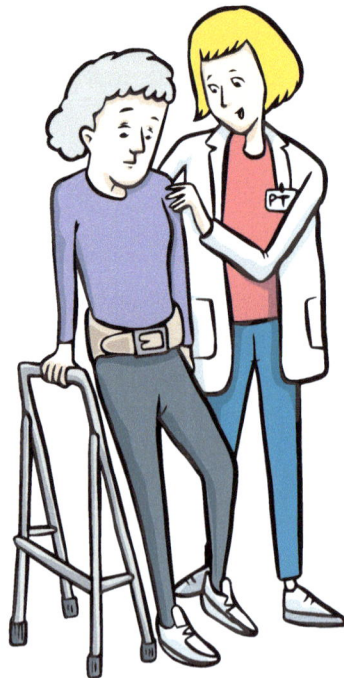

► Learn what help is needed while getting around in a wheelchair or when walking with a walker or cane.

Occupational Therapist (OT):

plans treatment and special equipment needed to help the person become as independent as he can.

These include self-care skills such as bathing, grooming, dressing, making meals and eating. The OT treats visual-perceptual skills (how the brain interprets what the eyes see) and hand and arm use. He or she also provides splints for positioning weak limbs.

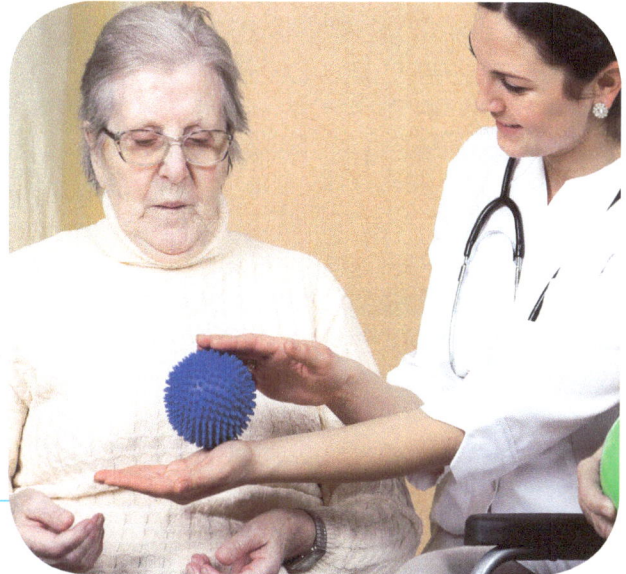

Physical Therapist (PT):

plans treatment needed to improve flexibility, strength, balance, coordination and endurance.

The PT teaches skills and provides equipment needed for safe transfers (moving from one place to another), relearning how to walk (gait training) or using a wheelchair.

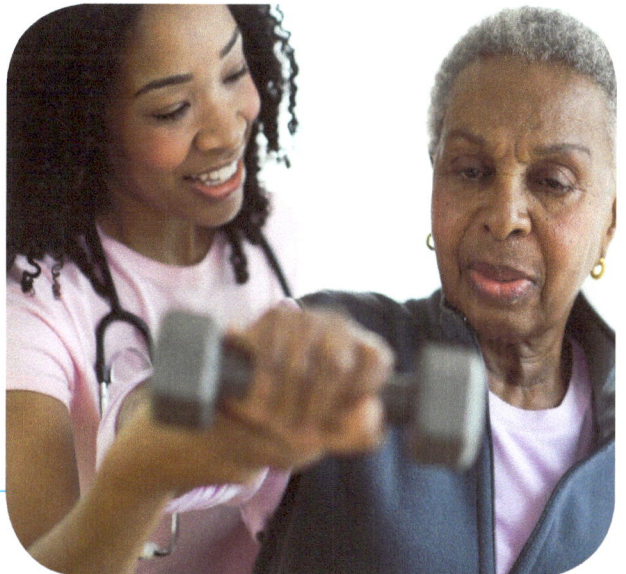

Communication

A stroke can cause a person to have trouble speaking, writing and/or understanding what words mean **(aphasia).**

Your loved ones may not understand that you can't come up with the right words to express your thoughts and feelings. This can be very hard on both of you, so be patient.

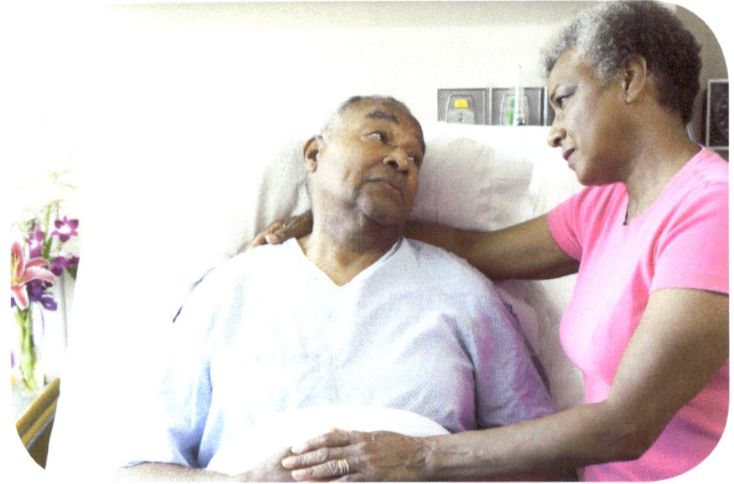

Family tips:

► Speak to your loved one in a normal tone. Just because he can't speak does not mean that he can't hear. If he did not have a hearing problem before his stroke, he most likely does not have one now.

► Don't talk as if the person isn't there. Even if he has trouble understanding, it's important that he feel included.

► Speak to him as an adult, but talk slowly, and use simple sentences. Shouting or talking in a noisy room makes it harder to understand.

► Use gestures along with words. If he has trouble speaking, ask him to point to what he needs.

► When you talk to him, be sure the person can see you. The look on your face and the way you move can help him understand.

► Ask short questions that can be answered with yes or no. Ask a question in more than one way to make sure he understands.

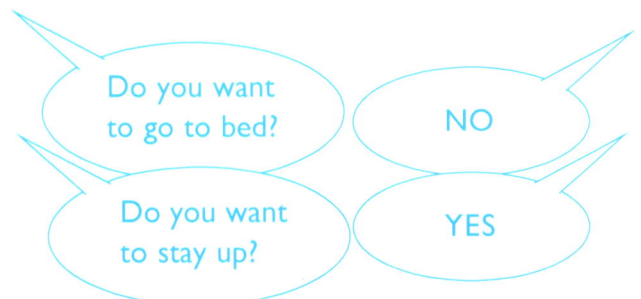

Do you want to go to bed?

NO

Do you want to stay up?

YES

Speech/language pathologist:

treats problems in communication, thinking skills and how the patient interacts with others.

He or she also assesses and treats swallowing problems that may occur during eating and drinking.

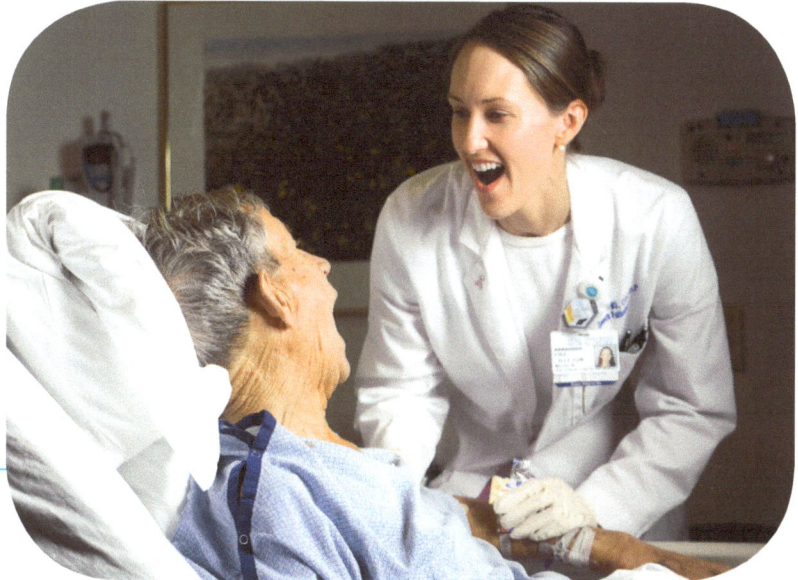

Eating, drinking & swallowing

A stroke can cause weakness and loss of feeling in the mouth, tongue and throat. Weak muscles can cause a person to choke or cough when eating or drinking. You may not be able to close your mouth in a normal way. You may drool or store food in the weak side of your mouth.

A special X ray **(modified barium swallow)** may be done to show the type of swallowing problem. This will give you a better idea of the kinds of food and liquids that can and cannot be swallowed safely.

Feeding may happen through a tube until you can swallow safely. The tube is placed through the nose and throat **(NG tube)** or straight into the stomach **(PEG tube).**

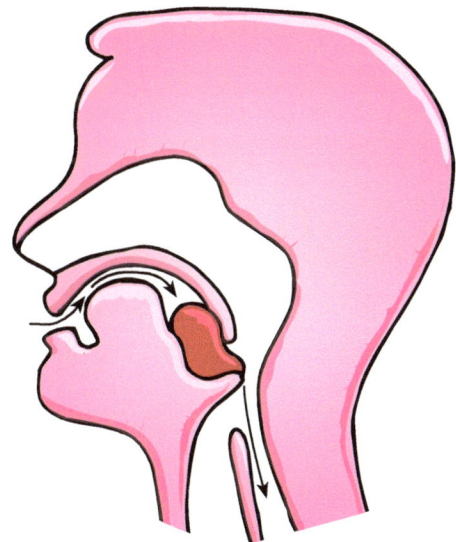

Helpful tips:

► If drooling is a problem, carry a handkerchief, and pat dry the weak side of your mouth. Let your loved ones remind you to do this until it happens naturally. Drooling often gets better with time.

► Before eating, sit with the best posture you can. (See page 31.) If you must stay in bed, raise the head of your bed to help with swallowing.

► Eat on your own as much as you are able. It may be messy and even a little embarrassing at first, but practice will make eating easier.

► A special diet may be needed for a while. You may need food cut into small pieces or creamed. Thick liquids such as milk shakes and puddings are often easier to swallow than water.

► An occupational therapist can give you special tools to make eating easier. These may be special knives, forks and spoons; mats that hold dishes in place; dishes that are built up for scooping, or cups that won't tip.

► Trust that you will get much better with time, practice and a LOT of patience.

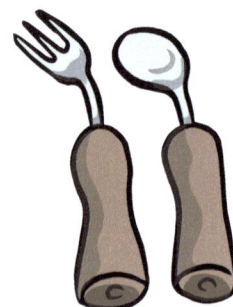

Family tips:

► At mealtime, make sure the room is quiet and still. Place food where it can be seen.

► Encourage your loved one to put food in the stronger side of his mouth. You may also need to remind him to take small bites and chew slowly. Teach him to pat his cheek after every few bites to check for food "pocketing".

Bladder & bowel function

People who have a stroke often "wet" or "soil" themselves. (Wetting is more common than soiling.) This loss of bladder or bowel control is called incontinence. The person may not know that he needs to relieve himself. Sometimes he may know but not be able to tell anyone.

Dealing with this is very hard for the person and others. Sometimes a tube (catheter) is put in the bladder to drain urine until he regains control.

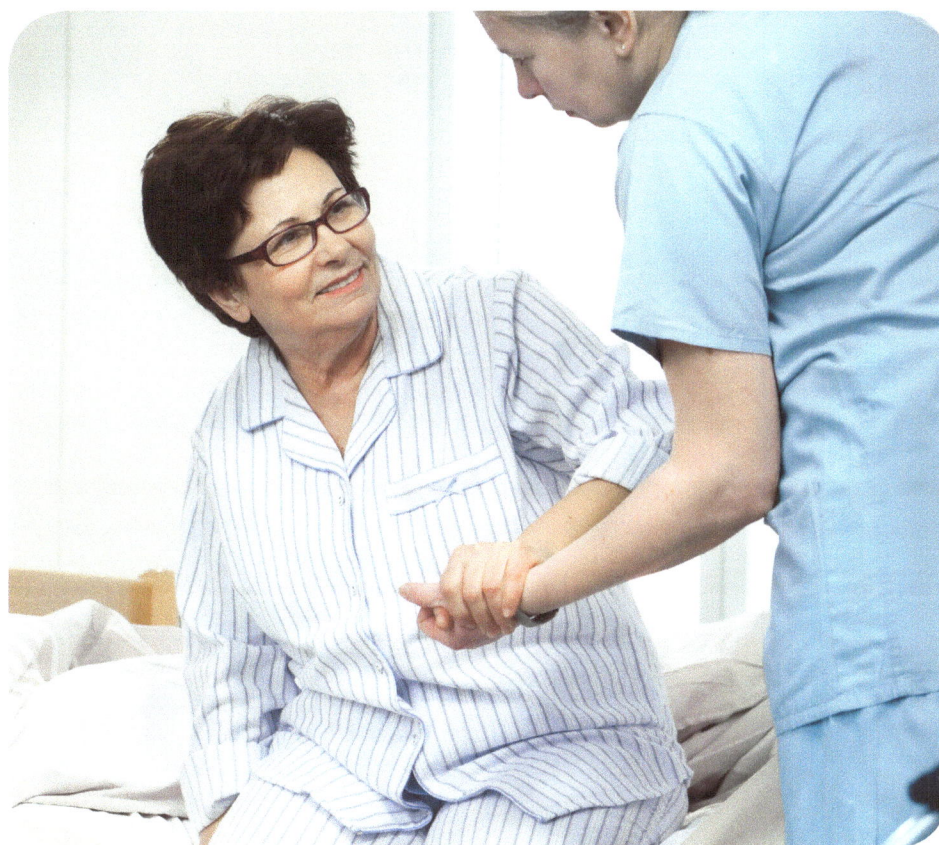

► If you can't speak, set up a signal to use to let someone know your needs.

► Try to urinate on a schedule such as every 2 to 3 hours. Include after meals, before sleeping and when you wake up.

► Keep skin clean and dry to help prevent an uncomfortable rash.

Senses (sight, touch, position)

People learn about the world around them through their senses. Two senses that often change after a stroke are touch and sight. A person may have trouble knowing if something is hot or cold. He may not notice when a sharp object touches his body. Also, he may not know what position his limbs are in without looking at them.

Blurred and double vision are also common after stroke. Blindness when looking to one side (visual field cut) can cause a person to fall or trip over things.

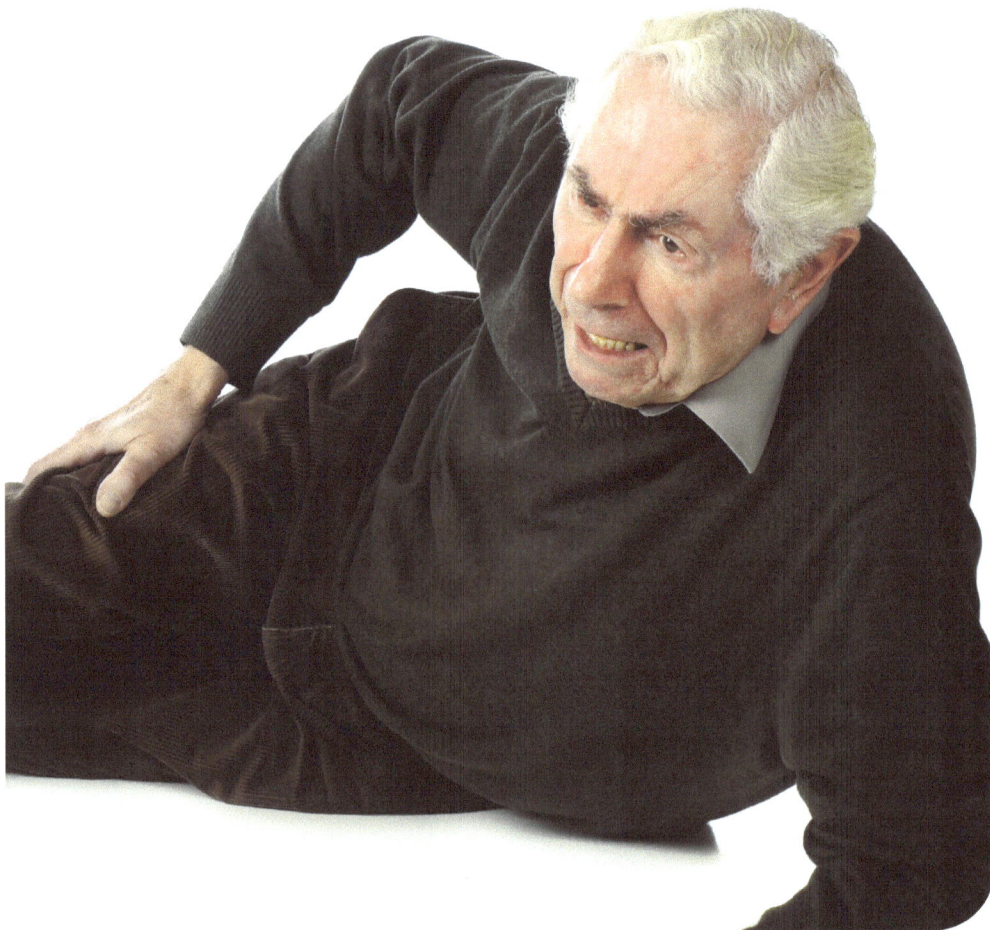

This is one type of visual field cut:

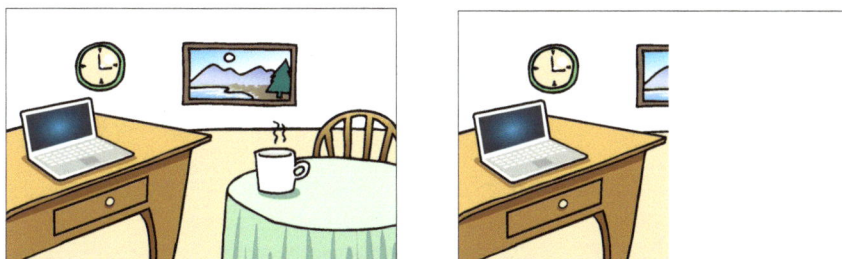

Because some of your senses have been damaged by the stroke, you must take extra safety measures. Discuss which ones you need to know about with your doctor and therapists.

Safety tips:

► Before moving from one place to another, look at how your arms and legs are positioned. If you need help, let someone put them in the right position before you move.

► Splints, braces and new shoes can irritate skin. Increase wearing time a little bit each day, and check skin often for red or dark places.

► Help prevent burns. Remember to test water temperature with your "good" hand (the one not affected by the stroke) before bathing.

► If you have a visual field cut, practice turning your head toward the blind side. This brings things into your field of vision. With practice, you will begin doing this automatically.

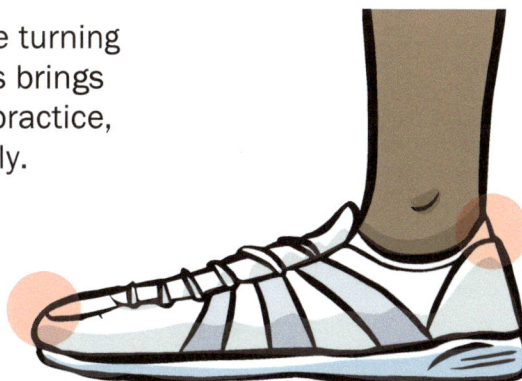

Behavior

Thoughts, feelings and actions almost always change after a stroke. Here are a few that may happen early in recovery.

Lability is a sudden outburst of emotion the person cannot control. After a stroke, a person may cry, laugh or become angry at odd times. This can frustrate and embarrass him.

Family tips:

► Remind everyone that lability is *caused* by the stroke.

► During an outburst, encourage him to stop and take a few deep breaths until he gains control.

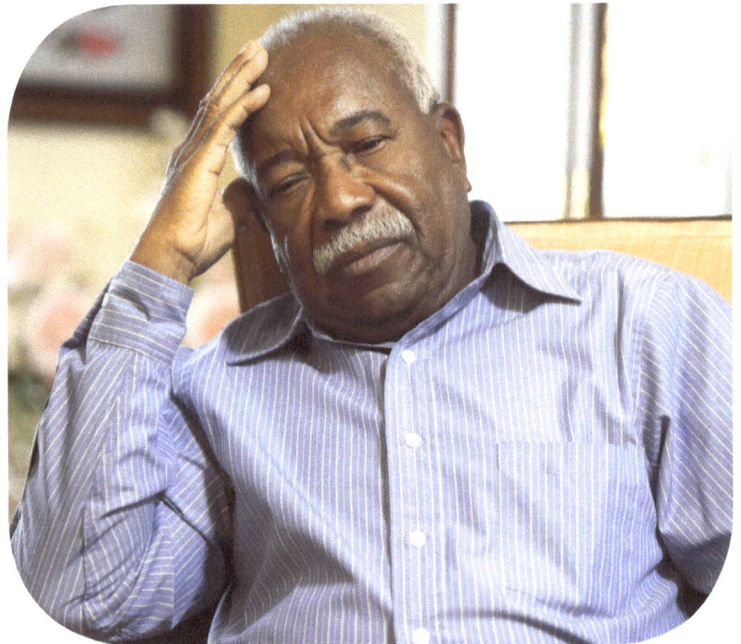

Depression is a long lasting feeling of deep sadness. Some strokes cause depression that needs to be treated with medicine. Tell the doctor if you notice these:

► unusual sadness

► poor appetite

► long crying spells

► more irritability

► can't sleep

Denial means you may not believe you have problems which are plain to others. This happens when a stroke harms the part of the brain that lets a person know that something about him has changed. Each person's awareness returns at its own rate. Even though it's hard, trust that your loved ones are being honest and are trying to help.

Family tips:

► Gently point out, "You did that differently before your stroke. Now you…"

► Keep your loved one safe until he can learn, in small stages, how he has changed. Most of the time denial goes away slowly as the person has problems doing things he knows he could do before the stroke.

Apraxia is trouble doing an activity even though there is strength and coordination to carry it out. The person knows what he wants to do and can do it when not thinking about it. But often he can't do the movements when he is asked to. For example, when trying to comb his hair he holds the comb upside down and moves it sideways.

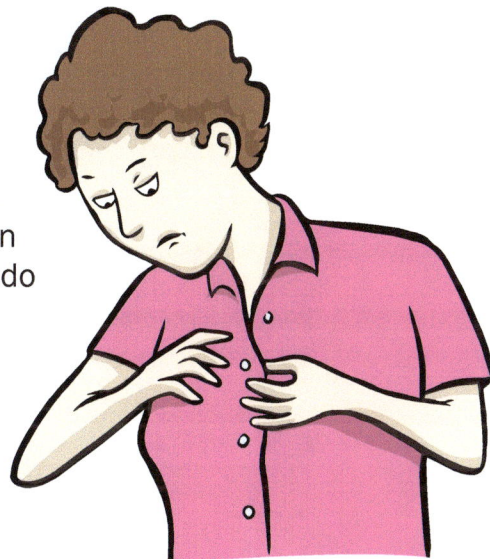

Family tips:

► Keep in mind that the person is not being stubborn when he doesn't do something that is asked of him.

► Talk through what you want him to do. Gently guide his hand or body, and show him what needs to be done.

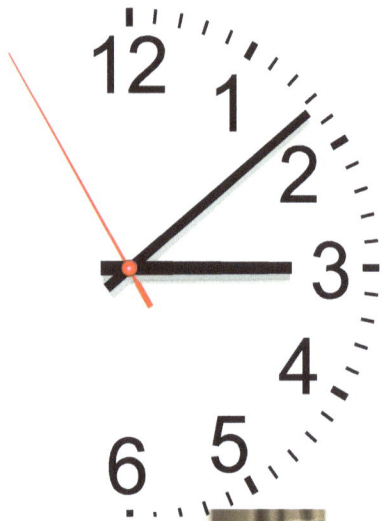

A stroke can change the ability to notice people or things on one side of the body. A person may **neglect** his own body on that side (often the left side). He may leave glasses hanging from one ear, eat from one side of the plate or leave pants down on one leg.

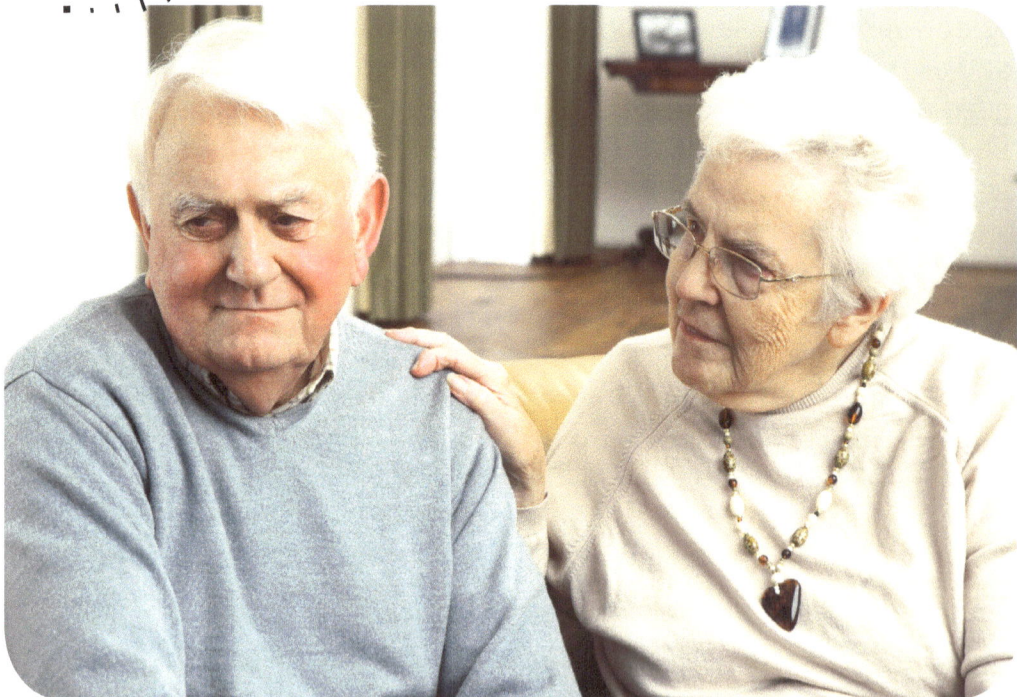

Family tips:

► Early in recovery, talk to the person from his normal side. Place things like food, glasses and telephone where he will notice them.

► As he becomes aware of this problem, begin to draw his attention to the side he neglects. Give him feedback about his progress.

Thinking

Strokes often cause **thinking problems.** At first, the person may be confused about who loved ones are and what has happened. Later, he may not be able to remember new things.

Helpful tips:

▶ If you are able to read, let someone prepare a notebook or electronic tablet for you. Include sections or download easy apps for:

- daily schedule
- notes about what goes on each day
- personal facts such as birthdays, phone numbers and addresses
- to-do list with reminders and alarms

▶ Ask for hints and choices when trying to remember things.

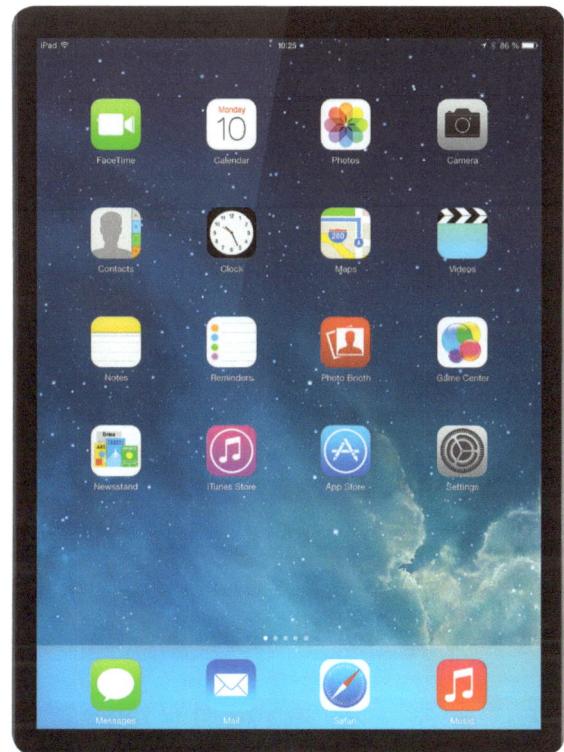

It's often hard to **pay attention** after a stroke. A person may not notice what is going on around him, or his attention span may be very short. He may be distracted or pulled away by noises, movement or his own thoughts.

Sometimes a person becomes **impulsive** (acts before thinking). He may move quickly without taking safety measures (like standing up before locking wheelchair brakes). Or he may suddenly shout something at a stranger.

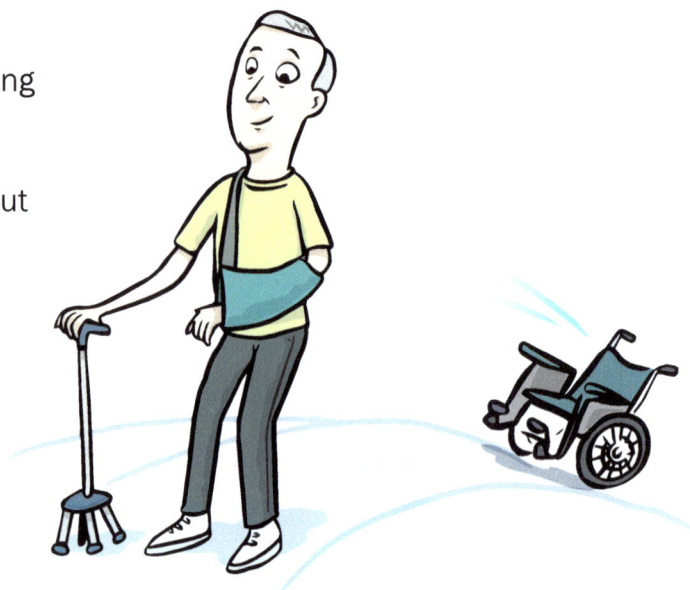

⊘ Helpful tips:

► Trust others to help you. Remember to:

1. STOP.   2. THINK.   3. DO IT SLOWLY.

Family tips:

► At first, you may have to guard the person's safety and not expect him to be aware of his actions. Choose a time when he is calm to teach him about thinking before acting.

► Keep activities short, and change them as attention fades. Slowly increase the amount of time spent on each task.

► Make the room quiet and still during activities. Focus on one activity instead of talking about other things while the patient is doing something.

Being safe and comfortable in bed...

While you are in bed (both in the hospital and later at home), you may need help changing positions every two hours. Blood flows better when weight is shifted off of a part of the body. This also helps prevent pressure ulcers (bedsores). Towel rolls, pillows and splints can keep weak limbs from becoming swollen, stiff or sore.

► Let someone close to you help the nurses look for red or dark, tender skin. Look under bony areas such as back of head, shoulders, hips, elbows, tailbone and heels.

► Keep skin clean and dry.

► Avoid dragging a weak body part across sheets. This can tear tender skin.

► Learn how to put on splints. Keep a list of times when they should be worn.

► Keep bed clean and free of crumbs, lumps and wrinkles.

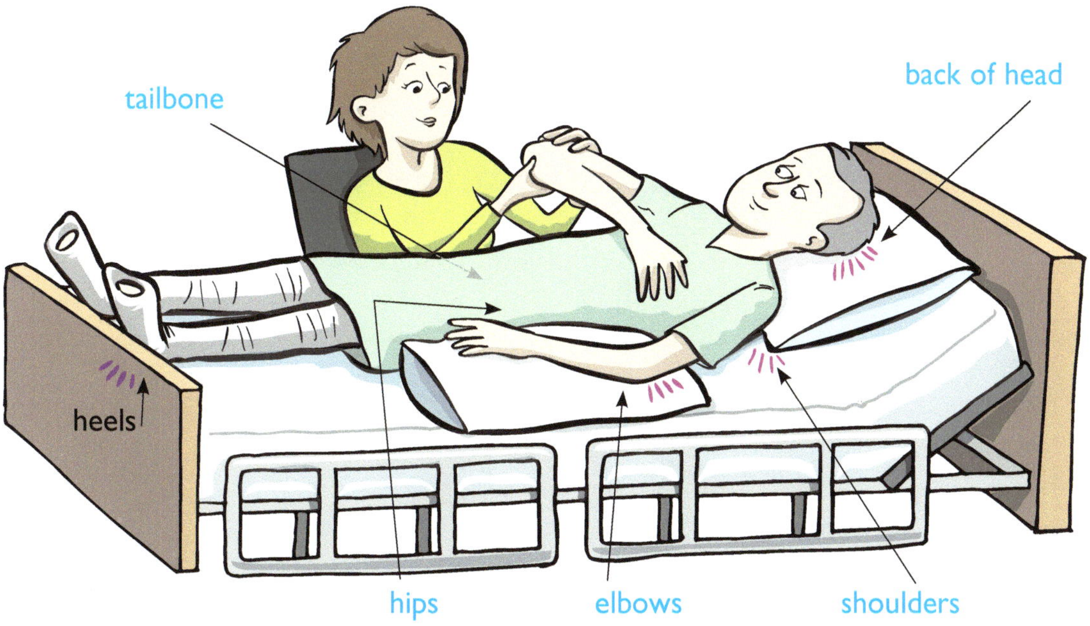

tailbone

back of head

heels

hips   elbows   shoulders

These are good positions while in bed:

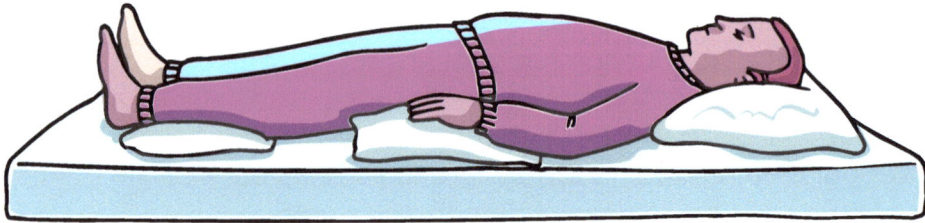

Flat on back

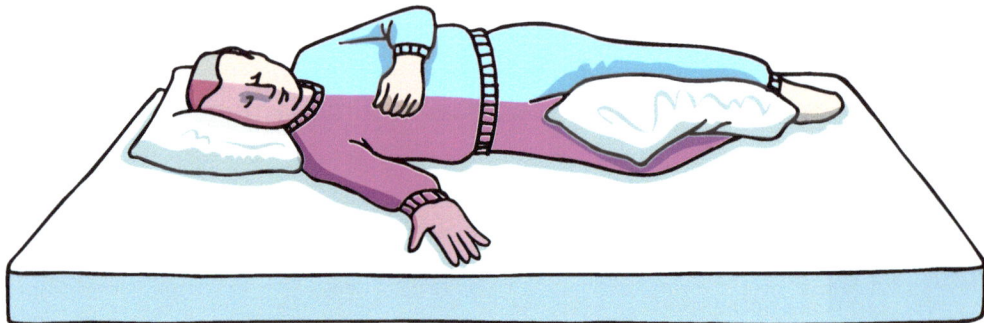

Lying on weak side

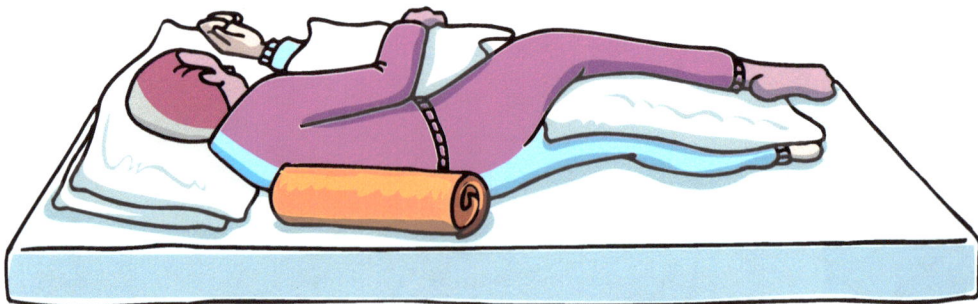

Lying on strong side

...and Out of Bed

Good sitting posture is very important during recovery from stroke. It helps improve balance and the person's awareness of himself and things around him. Good posture makes it easier and safer to move weak limbs. It can also make a weak voice sound louder and help prevent choking while eating.

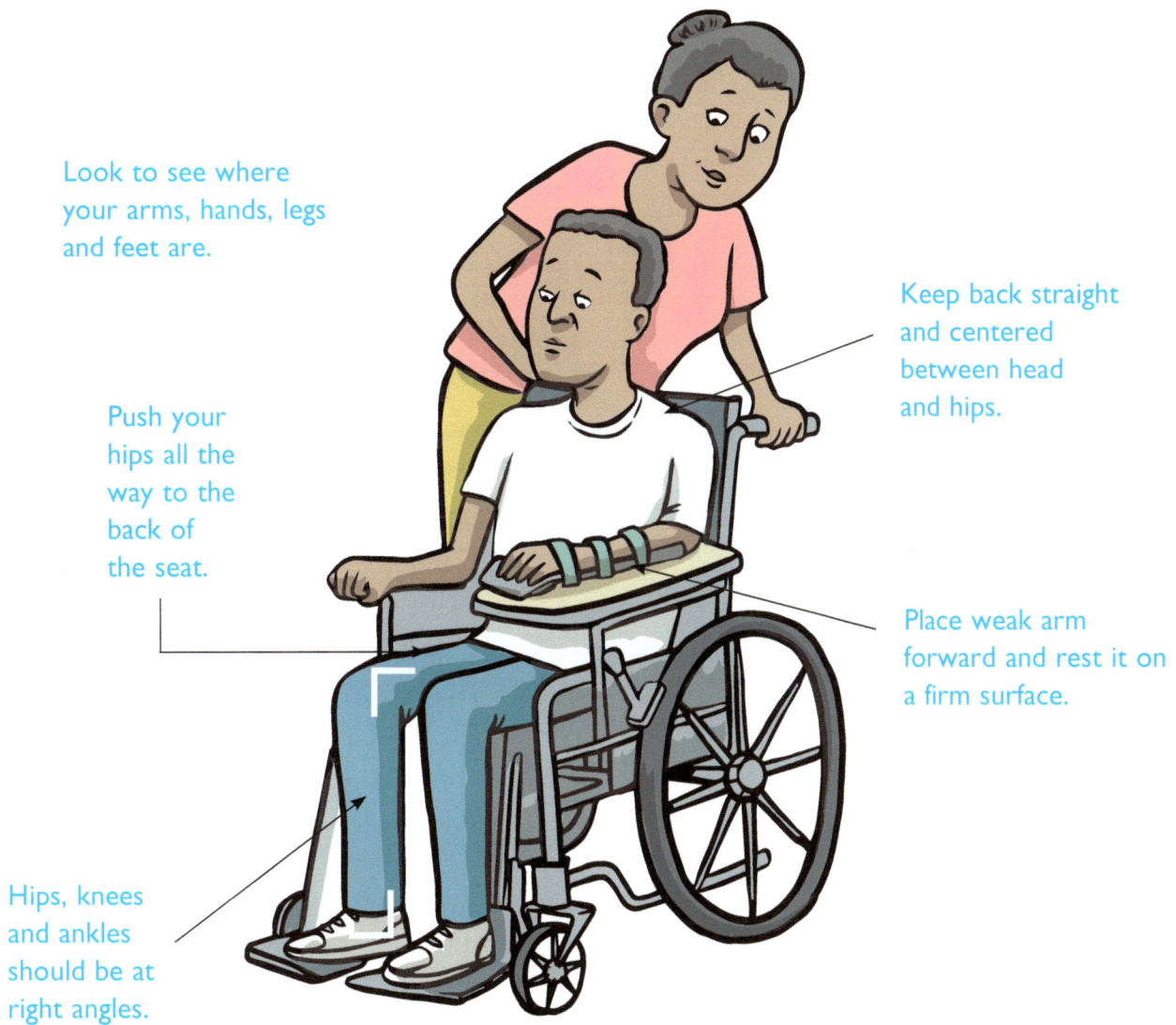

Look to see where your arms, hands, legs and feet are.

Push your hips all the way to the back of the seat.

Hips, knees and ankles should be at right angles.

Keep back straight and centered between head and hips.

Place weak arm forward and rest it on a firm surface.

Moving Around

Learning how to move from one place to another (**transfer**) is important for both your helper's safety and yours. The physical or occupational therapist (see page 17) can teach you how to move from the chair, bed, toilet, tub and car.

If you use a wheelchair, you will need to learn:

► how to use the moveable chair parts and brakes

► the best position for the wheelchair and the place you're moving toward

► the best position for your body and your helper's body before you begin the transfer and during the movement

► what to do if you fall

It's a good idea to talk about what you are doing just before the transfer. Allow someone to help with just what you need to stay safe. Learn the best way to transfer so you can teach others.

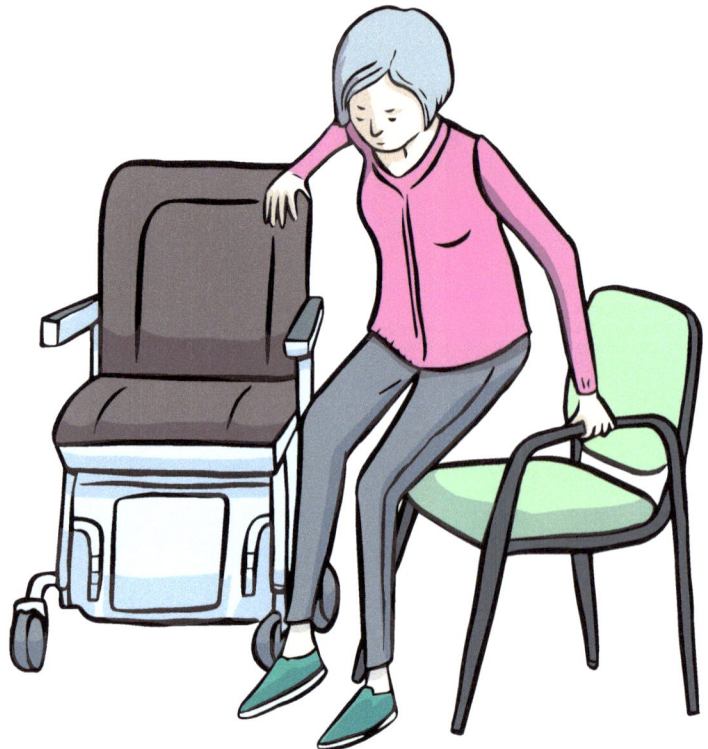

Understanding Your Feelings

Grief

Feelings of grief are common among people whose lives have been affected by a loss such as sudden or chronic illness. Grief can last from days to months, and it can involve many phases. Each person grieves in his or her own way. You and your loved ones may or may not go through the phases listed here.

You may feel frustrated and guilty about your feelings as you adjust to changes in your life and in those you love. Your feelings are OK. You may move back and forth between the phases of grief during recovery and long after therapy ends.

As you go through grief, talk with people you trust. Talking can bring comfort and relief.

The first phase of grief is **denial.** Common statements during this time may sound like:

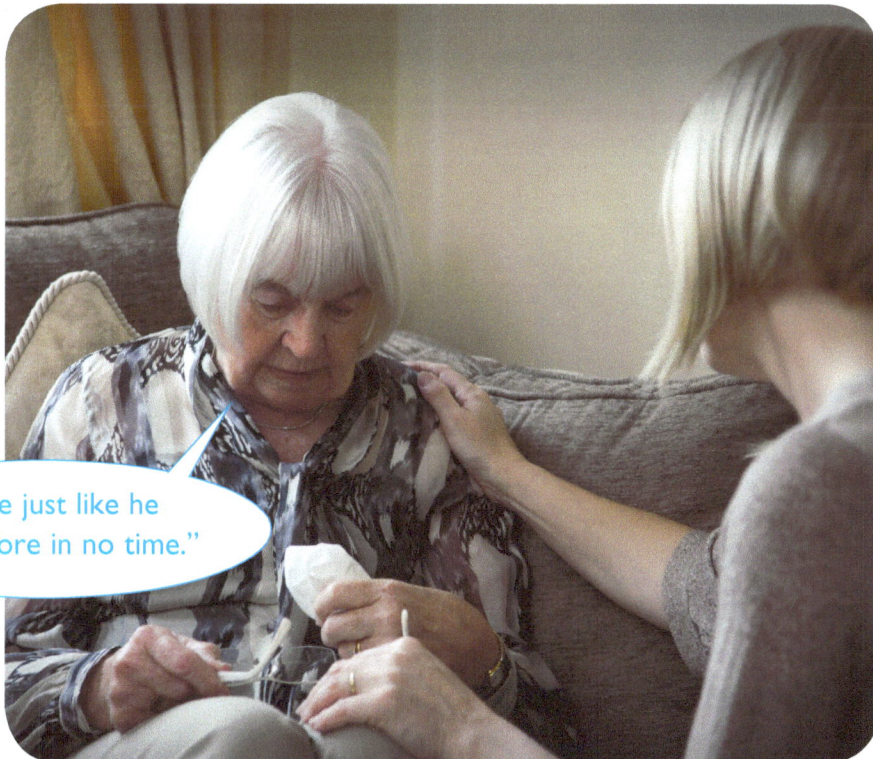

"He'll be just like he was before in no time."

Next, you may become angry and frustrated. These feelings are often focused on the health team, other family members or even yourself. **Anger** may be expressed like this:

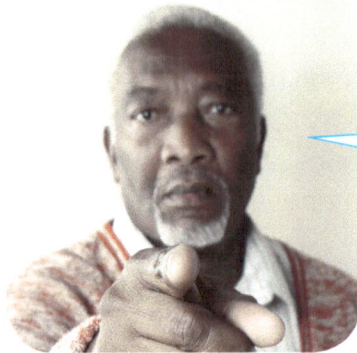

"The doctor is just trying to confuse us. If the nurse was doing her job, she wouldn't be like this."

Bargaining with a Higher Power is also common during the grief process. You may have thoughts such as:

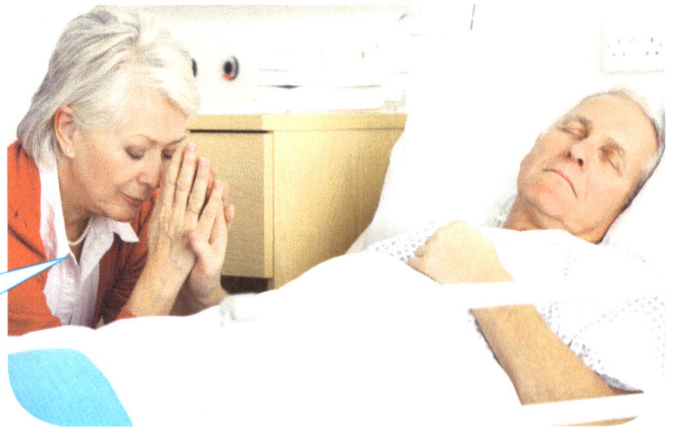

"God, if you'll just make him well, I'll never _____ again."

The next stage may be the most painful, but it's a big step toward coping with your feelings. It is **depression.** Besides feeling sad, helpless and hopeless, you may withdraw from those close to you and stop taking care of yourself. Loss of sleep and appetite are common. You can work through this phase by expressing your sadness and listening to the support you receive. During this stage, people sometimes say:

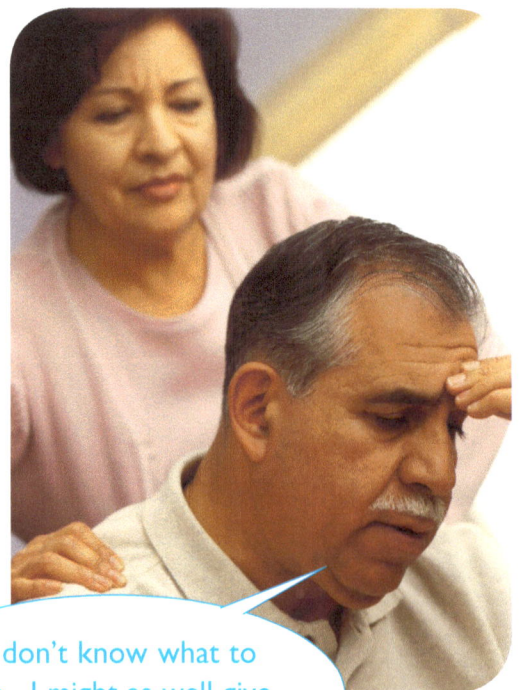

"I don't know what to do— I might as well give up. Why bother?"

You will start to feel better as you enter the next phase and begin to accept the changes in your life and in those you love. Yes, your life has changed. You can't change what has happened, but you can accept the challenge of this new life. **Acceptance** may sound like this:

"Since this is how things are now, I'm going to handle it this way…"

"My family and friends need me, and I need to get back into the swing of things."

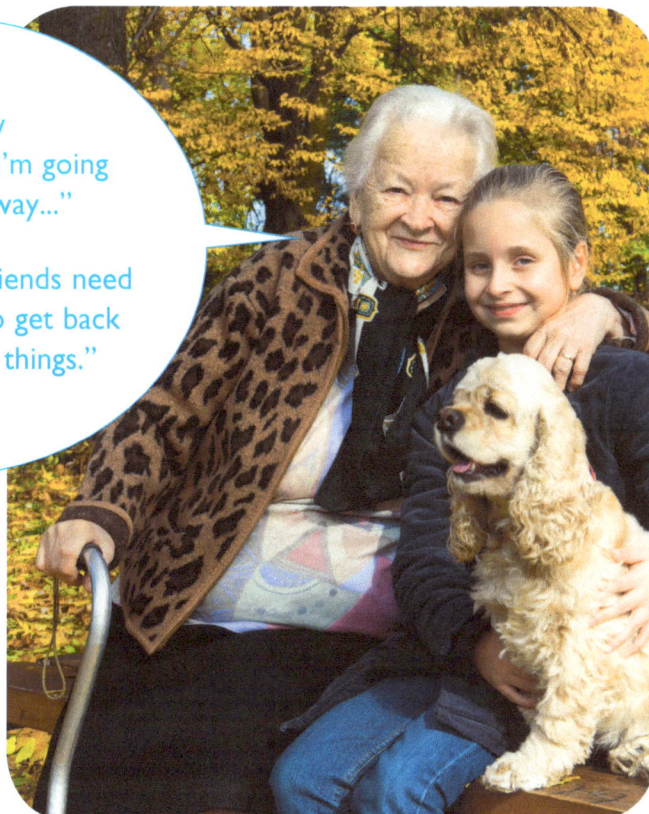

⊙ **Helpful tips:**

► For now, try to accept the changes in your life. Turn your hopes into goals, and take small steps to reach each goal.

► Celebrate each bit of progress.

► Talk with others who have been touched by a stroke. You may be surprised to find that they share your feelings. Such talk may bring you comfort.

► Ask those close to you how they are coping. Remind them to take time to do things themselves to stay healthy. Encourage them to do something relaxing–go for a walk, play a sport, exercise in a gym, listen to soothing music or take a warm bath. Feeling refreshed helps everyone think clearly and have patience during stressful times.

► Call or visit online some of the resources in the back of this book (see pages 47 and 48). They are good sources of information about stroke. They can also put you in touch with local support groups and other family members of stroke survivors.

► Be willing to seek professional help during these grief phases.

► Talk with children often about their day-to-day lives and feelings. You can learn how they cope by seeing changes in their outlook and how they act.

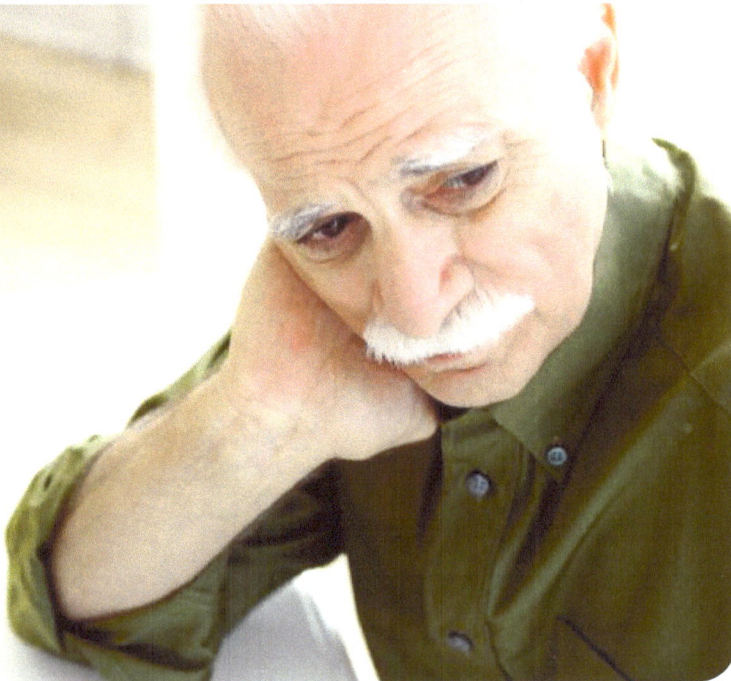

Some strokes harm the part of the brain that controls mood. Some people who have had a stroke may need medical care to help with anger, anxiety or depression. Feelings of deep sadness may not stop until the person gets the right medicine (anti-depressant). A doctor or psychologist can help you get the right help for mood changes.

Leaving the Hospital

There is a lot to learn before you go home or to another facility.

Ask a family member to go with you to all therapies at least once so they can learn how to assist you. Ask the health team to write instructions for care, and practice them before discharge. Use the list on the next page to help with instructions.

Give yourself time to adjust to being home, and try to limit the number of visitors at first. Try to avoid busy public places during your first few outings. It may take awhile to adjust to changes and you may tire easily.

Choose a health professional whom you trust to discuss changes in sexual activity.

Family tips:

▶ Your loved one needs to gain as much independence as he can, so help him only with what is needed.

▶ Learn about any changes needed to the home such as building a ramp or adding handrails to stairs and bathrooms.

▶ If you need help at home, plan to have a number of caregivers. Both caregivers and the patient need breaks from each other to stay "fresh".

▶ Stick to a daily routine at home. Post a schedule where all can see it.

Ask the health team which of these activities you need to learn before leaving the hospital. Take photos of equipment you may need later and jot down lots of notes.

Activities of Daily Living (ADL's)

Medicine — names of drugs, purpose, amount, times taken, side effects

Exercises — exercises to help with thinking and movement and how often to do them

Using Equipment — how to adjust and use equipment, who to call for repairs

Transfers — how to get in and out of bed, tub, car, on and off the toilet and up from the floor

Walking — how to help with balance, reminders needed when walking over different surfaces, curbs and stairs

Grooming and Dressing — hints before bathing and dressing to help increase independence and confidence

Eating — safety tips for swallowing, types of foods to avoid

Toileting — how to set up a schedule, how to give and accept the right amount of help

Behavior — what to expect, who and when to call for help

Communication — best methods, how much help to give

Sexual Activity — how to deal with physical changes, comfortable positions, other ways to show affection

Enjoying Life

It's important to stay active after a stroke. Activity helps the body heal and keeps spirits up for the stroke survivor and the family. With a few changes or special equipment, you can safely enjoy:

► hobbies

► visits to church, restaurants, friends

► exercise

► sexual activity

► chores around the house

► returning to work or volunteer activities

A recreational therapist can help you explore new hobbies and leisure activities in your community. An assistive technology specialist may help you get special equipment for speaking, driving, or other daily activities. Check with a nearby college or hospital to learn what is available in your area.

Ask the healthcare team to help you find local support group meetings for you and your family.

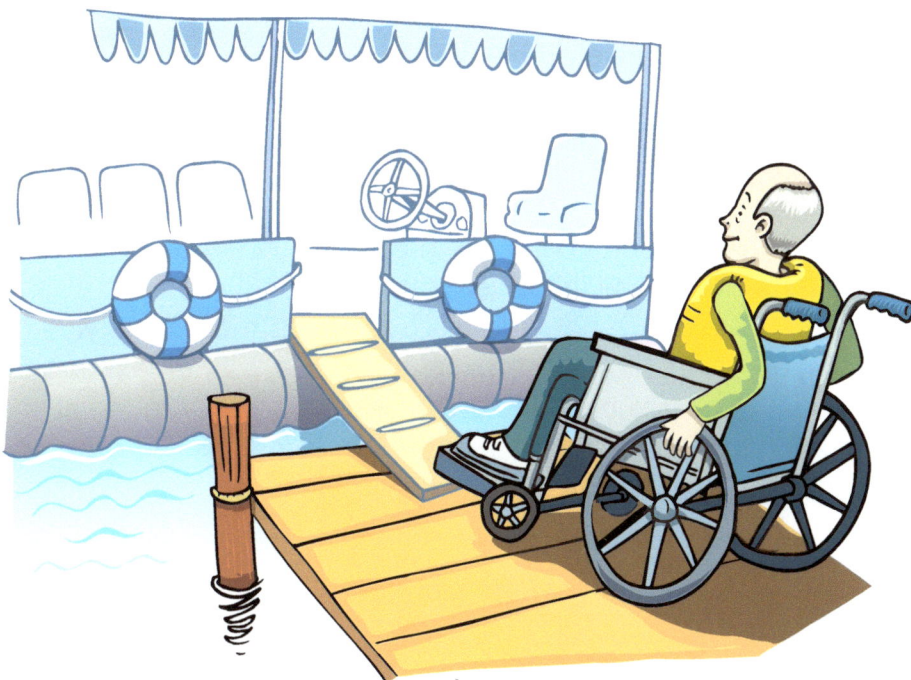

Choosing the Best Care After Discharge

You may still face physical, communication, thinking and/or behavior challenges when it's time to leave the hospital.

Talk to your hospital service coordinator about places that give the type of care you need now and as your needs change. The best choice will depend on patient and family needs as well as finances.

Insurance covers different types of care, but must be approved first. Service coordinators can help by asking your insurance carrier to approve the care you need next.

Types of care

► **An acute rehabilitation (therapy) facility** can be in a hospital or separate facility. Patients stay overnight for therapy and medical care from nurses and doctors each day. They need to be strong enough for 3 hours of therapy, 5 days a week.

► **A skilled nursing facility or nursing home** both provide therapy and nursing services, but for less time than an acute rehabilitation facility. Therapy is 1-2 hours a day for 3-5 days each week. These services are often covered by insurance for a short time. But if you need care for a long time, coverage by private insurance or government programs may be limited.

► **Home health care** can be given in the home for those whose improvements are slow and who are not able to go to a treatment facility. Speech, occupational and physical therapies, as well as nursing and social work, are provided 1-3 times per week. A nursing assistant can offer personal support with activities like bathing, dressing and staying safe.

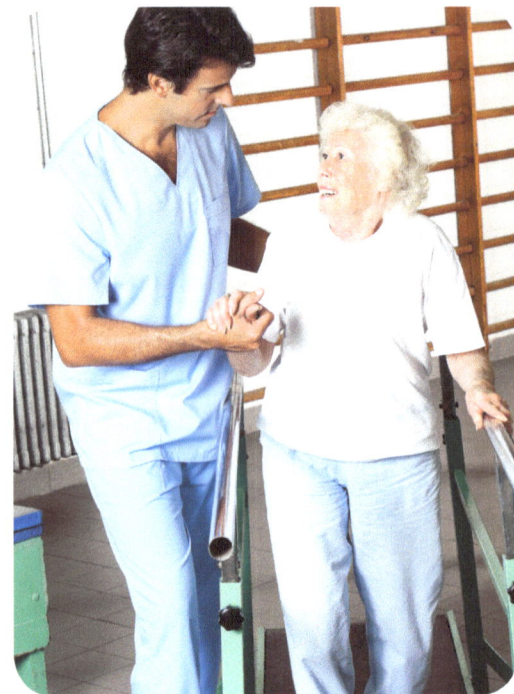

► **Outpatient facilities**
provide therapies at a clinic if you are able to leave your home. They have special tools and machines that therapists can use to help you regain your strength and abilities. These services usually happen 2-3 times a week.

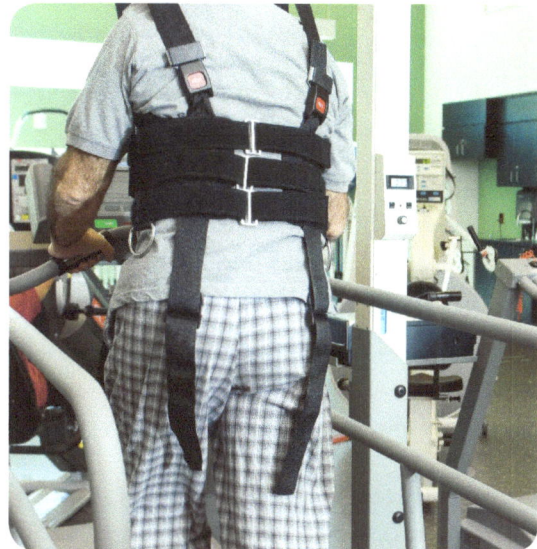

► **Living at home**
or in the home of a relative is often chosen for financial reasons or because there is someone who can take care of the person's needs. It is helpful to have several family members, neighbors and friends pitch in to create a strong circle of support.

► **Respite care**
can bring much needed relief to families caring for loved ones at home. Respite is usually provided by helpers in the home but sometimes in a nursing facility for short periods to give the caregiver a break.

► **Assisted living communities**
offer a range of support like personal care, therapy, help with medication, meals and shopping. This is a good choice if you lived alone before the stroke but may now need a little more daily help. Medical insurance doesn't usually pay for this, but long-term care policies may.

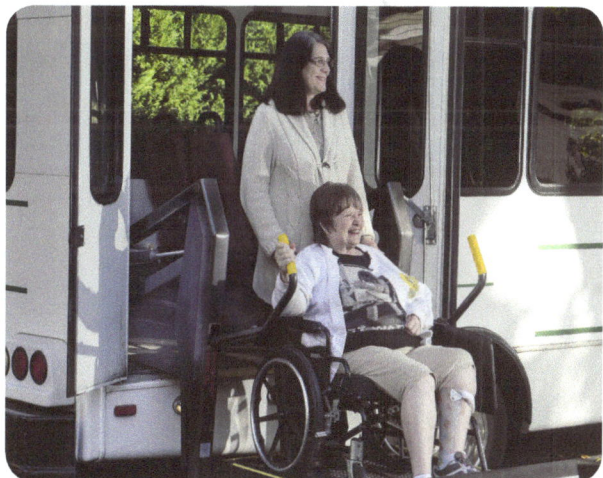

► **Local senior service agencies and statewide independent living centers** offer resources for transportation, housing, home care, wheelchair ramps, companionship and many more needs. In some areas, these resources are free or low-cost to those in financial need.

The Road to Recovery

Whether your care happens at home or in a live-in center, the road to recovery has just begun. It can be a long, hard road with many forks and turns. There will be joy during good days and frustration on the hard days. You may not be able to feel, see or do things as you did before the stroke. There is almost always a need for more therapy. Someone from the hospital may call to check on you after discharge. Be sure to report progress or any new problems you may be having.

Whatever choices you make now, know that things will change in time. The care you need may change. You may need a different plan as family needs or finances change. Keep looking ahead, while being pleased with how you are doing now.

Most of all, congratulations! You've made it through the most critical time of recovery and are on your way to the next phase.

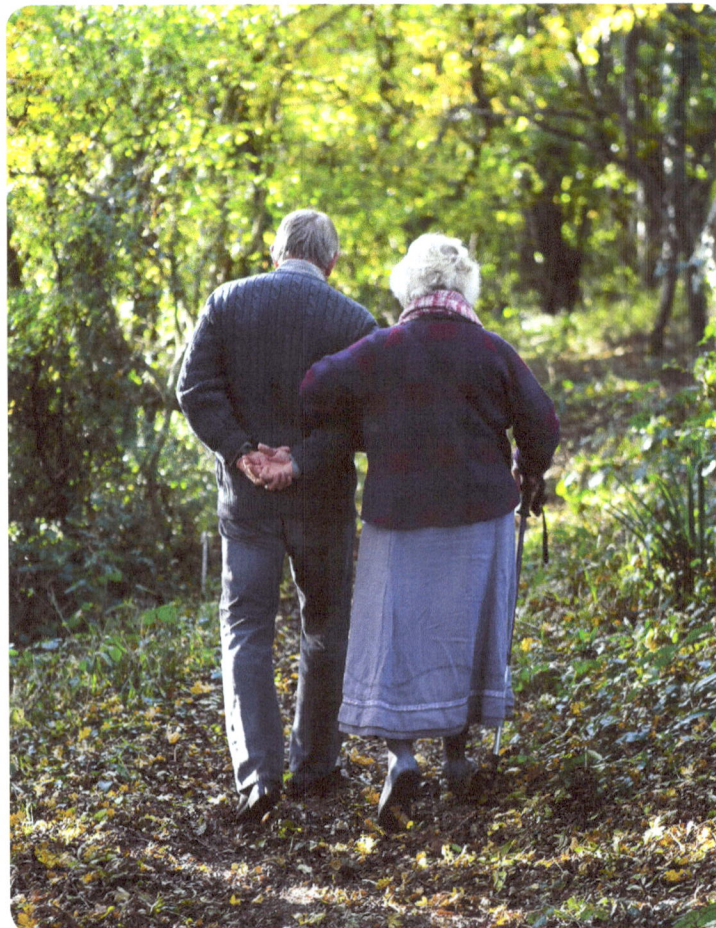

Brain diagrams

Ask the health team to use these drawings when talking with you about stroke.

Brain seen from side

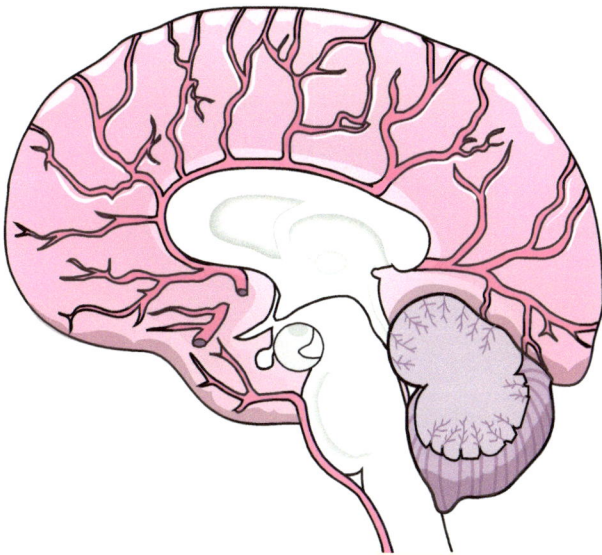

Brain seen from below

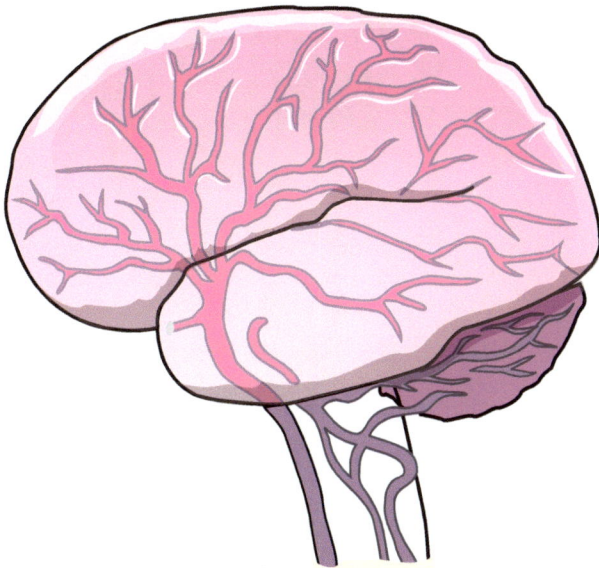

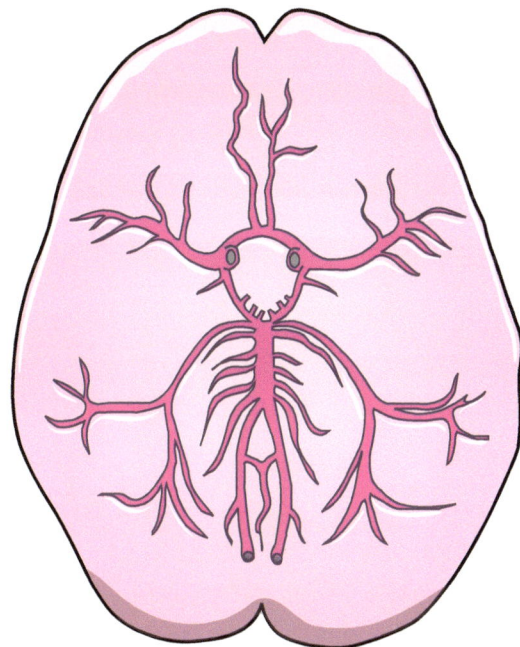

Preventing Stroke

It's time to think of steps you can take to prevent another stroke. Take a look at the risk factors. Some cannot be changed, but some can. If you need to change your diet, a registered dietitian can give great tips on how to make those changes and still enjoy the foods you love.

Risk Factors You Can't Change:

▶ **Age older than 55**
As we age our risk for stroke increases.

▶ **Race**
African Americans have the highest rate of stroke.

▶ **Family history**
You are at risk for stroke if someone in your family has had a stroke or heart disease.

▶ **Prior stroke**
Your risk for stroke is greater if you've already had one.

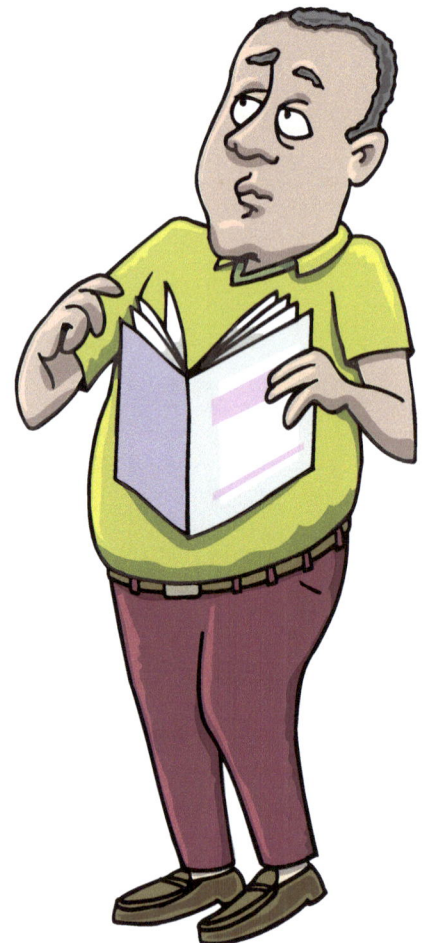

The Ones You Can Control:

► **High blood pressure**
Check your blood pressure often. If you have high blood pressure, take your medicines as your doctor tells you, even if you feel well.

► **Heart disease**
Follow your doctor's advice and take medicines as prescribed.

► **Diabetes**
Keep your blood sugar under control. People with diabetes are more likely to develop blood clots that cause strokes. Watch your diet, take medicines as prescribed, and exercise regularly.

► **Smoking**
If you smoke, quit. Smoking makes your blood vessels narrow. This makes it harder for blood to get to your brain. Even long-time smokers lower their risk for stroke by quitting.

► **Obesity**
Overweight people are more likely to have high blood pressure, heart disease, high cholesterol and diabetes. Reaching your ideal body weight and exercising will reduce your risk for stroke and other diseases.

► **High cholesterol**
Have your cholesterol checked, try to lower the fat in your diet, and take your medicines as your doctor tells you.

Control 3 Risk Factors At Once

• Heart Disease

• Obesity

• High Cholesterol

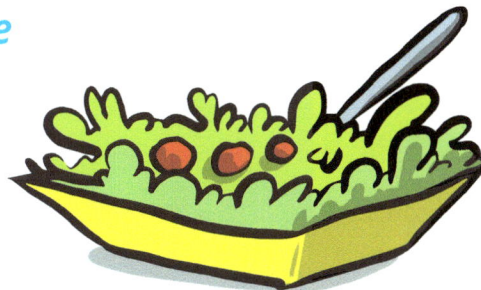

Studies show that eating **more** fruits, vegetables and grains and **fewer** meats and fats can help you do this.

A Word About Seizures

A small number of people have seizures after a stroke. A seizure happens when faulty electrical signals from the brain change the way a body functions. Knowing what to do in advance can make you feel more secure and help your loved ones keep you safe.

Some seizures are mild and may cause a person to stare into space and have a blank expression for a short time. Others may cause muscles on one side of the body to twitch or jerk.

A "generalized" seizure is stronger and makes muscles in the whole body become stiff and have a repeated jerking movement. It is normal for a person to be confused and tired for a while after this type of seizure.

If you think you may have had a seizure, let your doctor know right away. Don't drive a car until your doctor says it's ok.

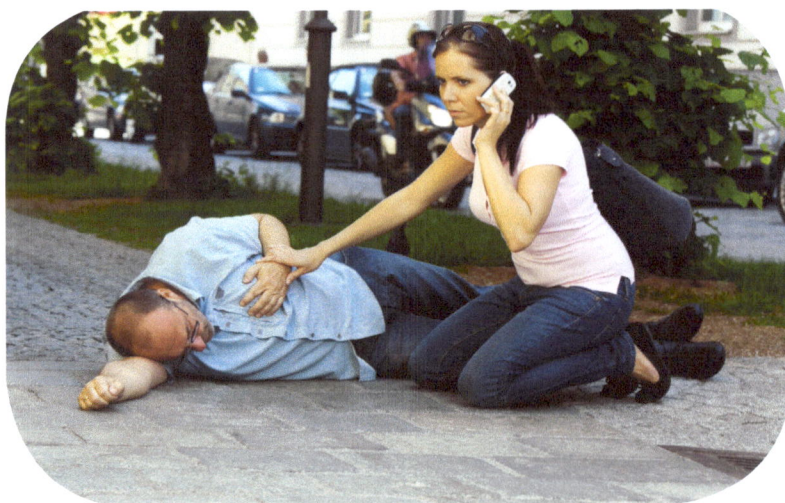

Family tips:

► Try to turn the person having a seizure on his side, and put something soft under his head. Reassure him that everything is ok.

► Don't put anything in his mouth—he will not swallow his tongue.

► Call 911 if the seizure lasts longer than 3 minutes or if the person has trouble breathing.

► Stay with him, and call the doctor once the seizure stops. After testing, a medication may be given to help prevent other seizures.

Resources

For more reading material, listings of support groups and other information contact:

- **National Stroke Association**
  9707 East Easter Lane, Suite B
  Centennial, CO 80112
  800-STROKES or 800-787-6537
  stroke.org
  email: info@stroke.org

- **American Heart Association/ American Stroke Association**
  888-4-STROKE or 888-478-7653
  heart.org
  strokeassociation.org

- **Brain Aneurysm Foundation**
  888-272-4602
  bafound.org
  email: office@bafound.org

- **Brain Injury Association**
  1-800-444-6443
  biausa.org

- **National Rehabilitation Information Center**
  1-800-346-2742
  naric.com
  email: naricinfo@heitechservices.com

- **American Stroke Foundation**
  americanstroke.org
  913-649-1776

- **National Aphasia Association**
  aphasia.org
  email: naa@aphasia.org

- **Commission for Accreditation of Rehabilitation Facilities (CARF)**
  888-281-6531
  carf.org

Check with your hospital or doctor (health care provider) for local support groups.

More Resources

► **National Institute of Neurological Disorders and Stroke (NINDS)**
800-352-9424
ninds.nih.gov

► **Well Spouse Association**
800-838-0879
wellspouse.org
(Support for spouses
of the chronically ill)

► **Brain Injury Resource Center**
206-621-8558
www.headinjury.com
email: brain@headinjury.com

► **Caring Bridge**
caringbridge.org
Connects family and friends
throughout a health crisis.

► **My Stroke of Insight—A Brain Scientist's Personal Journey**
Jill Bolte Taylor, PhD
Viking Penguin, 2008

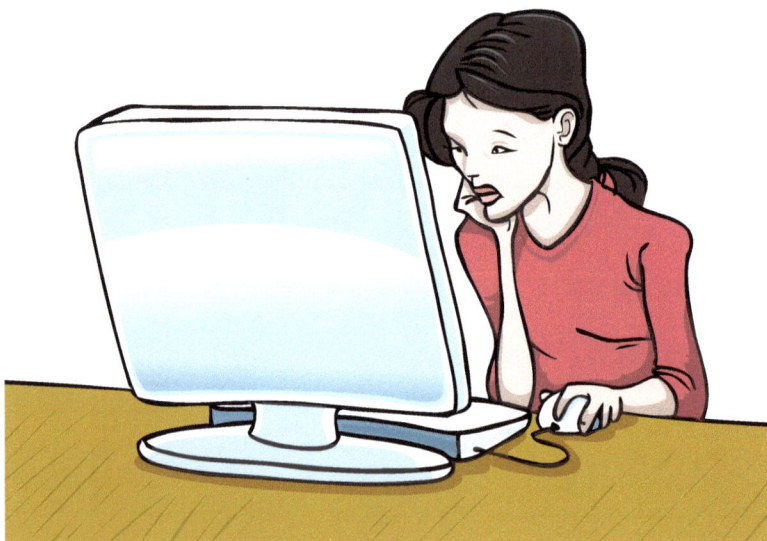

Dear Reader—

Knowing what to expect with a stroke can ease your stress and speed recovery. We hope this book has helped to do that for you. If you have any questions not answered here—**ask.** Ask your doctor, nurse or other members of your health care team. You can draw or make notes in this book and share the information with your family.

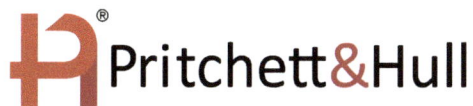

Pritchett&Hull

PRITCHETT & HULL ASSOCIATES, INC.
bringing Patients & Health together since 1973

Limited list of topics include:

Cardiac cath	Diabetes	Nutrition
Angioplasty	Traumatic brain injury	Hip and knee replacement
Heart surgery	Brain surgery	Chronic lung disease
Pacemaker	Kidney failure	
Exercise		

Write or call toll-free for a free catalog of all products and prices at 1-**800-241-4925** or visit P&H online at **www.p-h.com**